EVEN IF YOU'RE BROKEN

ESSAYS ON SEXUAL ASSAULT AND #METOO

EVEN IF YOU'RE BROKEN

ESSAYS ON SEXUAL ASSAULT AND #METOO

KATIE ROSE GUEST PRYAL

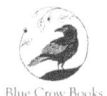

Blue Crow Books

Copyright © 2019 by Katie Rose Guest Pryal
All rights reserved.
No part of this book may be reproduced in any form or by any electronic or mechanical means, including information storage and retrieval systems, without written permission from the author, except for the use of brief quotations in a book review.

Publisher's Cataloging-in-Publication Data
Pryal, Katie Rose Guest. 1976-.
Even If You're Broken: Essays on Sexual Assault and #MeToo / Katie Rose Guest Pryal
p.____ cm.____
ISBN 978-1-947834-42-2 (Pbk.) | 978-1-947834-43-9 (Ebook)
1. Rape. 2. Women—crimes against. 3. Autobiography. I. Title.
814'.6 | PCN 2019948639

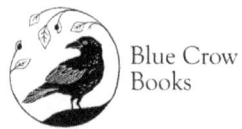

Blue Crow Books

Published by Blue Crow Books
an imprint of Blue Crow Publishing, LLC
Chapel Hill, NC
www.bluecrowpublishing.com
Cover photo by Stas Knop via Shutterstock
Cover Design by Lauren Faulkenberry
v.20200928

ALSO BY KATIE ROSE GUEST PRYAL

FICTION

Entanglement

Love and Entropy

Chasing Chaos

How to Stay

Fallout Girl

Take Your Charming Somewhere Else

NONFICTION

Life of the Mind Interrupted: Essays on Mental Health and Disability in Higher Education

We Are All Enemies of the State: And Other Essays on Speech

The Freelance Academic: Transform Your Creative Life and Career

Even If You're Broken: Essays on Sexual Assault and #MeToo

Praise for EVEN IF YOU'RE BROKEN

Rich in vulnerability and candor, Pryal's evocative essays remind us that the survivor journey is far from linear, and that there is power and beauty in our imperfect journey.

> ANDREA PINO, CO-AUTHOR OF *WE BELIEVE YOU: SURVIVORS OF CAMPUS SEXUAL ASSAULT SPEAK OUT*

A patchwork quilt of stories, raw emotion, and insights that will touch every reader. The result is moving, vital and somehow hopeful for survivors and society both.

> *WASHINGTON POST* BESTSELLING AUTHOR KELLY HARMS

Pryal deftly unpacks the way both individuals and institutions fail survivors—and clearly explains how we can all do better.

> BESTSELLING AUTHOR CAMILLE PAGÁN

A harrowing, necessary, and beautiful book.

KELLY J. BAKER, AWARD-WINNING AUTHOR OF
SEXISM ED: ESSAYS ON GENDER AND LABOR IN ACADEMIA

Praise for LIFE OF THE MIND INTERRUPTED

"Personal, political, polemical, and pointed in its vision for transforming higher education to be more inclusive of disabled and mentally ill people. ... If you want to understand how higher education is built, and not built, for people with disabilities—especially mental health–related ones—Pryal's book is for you."

BOOKRIOT

The advice and practical information makes this book a must read, not just for those in academia.

NEW YORK TIMES BESTSELLING AUTHOR KATE MORETTI FOR *BOOKTRIB MAGAZINE*

Pryal is one of the foremost writers of disability and higher education we have today.

> CATHERINE PRENDERGAST, AUTHOR OF
> *BUYING INTO ENGLISH: LANGUAGE AND INVESTMENT IN THE NEW CAPITALIST WORLD*

This is not a book to miss.

> KELLY J. BAKER, AWARD-WINNING AUTHOR OF
> *SEXISM ED: ESSAYS ON GENDER AND LABOR IN HIGHER EDUCATION*

These thoughtfully chosen and arranged essays grapple with issues relevant to disabled students and scholars as well as those who would be allies.

> KECIA ALI, AUTHOR OF *SEXUAL ETHICS AND ISLAM: FEMINIST REFLECTIONS ON QUR'AN, HADITH, AND JURISPRUDENCE*

Praise for THE FREELANCE ACADEMIC

A roadmap that's as practical as it is hopeful.

> BESTSELLING AUTHOR CAMILLE PAGÁN
> FOR *BOOKTRIB MAGAZINE*

Both a cautionary tale and a beacon of hope.

FOREWORD REVIEWS

So many academics—current, former, and struggling—will see themselves in Pryal's story. I hope just as many see all of the possibilities she enumerates, and understand, as she does, that the passions and talents that draw us to the university in the first place are often best used outside it.

REBECCA SCHUMAN, AUTHOR
OF SCHADENFREUDE, A LOVE STORY

With candor and vulnerability, Pryal shares her own experiences and hard-fought wisdom to make a compelling case for a rewarding professional life beyond the walls of traditional academia.

AMY IMPELLIZZERI, AWARD-WINNING NOVELIST
AND AUTHOR OF LAWYER
INTERRUPTED: SUCCESSFULLY
TRANSITIONING FROM THE PRACTICE OF
LAW—AND BACK AGAIN

A new, necessary book.

CATHERINE J. PRENDERGAST, AUTHOR OF
BUYING INTO ENGLISH: LANGUAGE AND
INVESTMENT IN THE NEW CAPITALIST
WORLD

CONTENTS

Content Warning	1
Introduction	3

PART I. THE PERSONAL

1. Why Birds Have Wings	15
2. Why I Didn't Report Being Raped	19
3. Being Counted	23
Reporting My Rape at a School Under Title IX Investigation	
4. Over Nothing	37
5. Even If You're Broken	44
6. Reading Romance When You Were Never a Virgin	50
7. Who's Kay?	60
8. Nightmare Room	80

PART II. THE PUBLIC

9. How to Write Publicly About Rape	113
10. Why Kesha Lost	121
11. Cosby and Rethinking Statutes of Limitations	132
12. Handling Institutional Atrocities	139
What We Can Learn from U.S. Gymnastics	
13. So Many Brett Kavanaughs	143

PART III. ON CAMPUS

14. How Campus Rape Changed Mental Health Privacy for All	151
15. Banning College Athletes for Sexual Violence Convictions Is Not Enough	166
16. Why We Should All Care About FERPA	172

17. Predatory Professors 186
18. MeToo Comes to Campus 196

Can We Stop Sexual Harassment in Higher Ed?

Notes 203
Acknowledgments 205
About the Author 209

For my gentle husband and sons

CONTENT WARNING

This is a book about sexual trauma and its aftereffects.
Some people, like me, who have suffered sexual trauma and continue to suffer its aftereffects need content warnings to allow us to fully engage with and appreciate our world.

The book contains stories and details of rape, sexual assault, sexual harassment, child sexual assault, and traumatic reactions to assault.

INTRODUCTION

I started *Even If You're Broken* in 2016. At the time, the book had a different title—a wittier, cuter title. By early 2016, I'd written and published enough on sexual assault, rape, and sexual harassment that I knew I could write a good book about these hard topics. The book would take personal stories, put them alongside research and reporting, and, with luck, change the world a little.

In the spring, I drafted a book proposal. I was feeling hopeful that the book would make a difference, that it would carry forward the work that so many of us had been doing, work on Title IX, for example, holding universities accountable and changing laws, creating an environment in which survivors felt safer coming forward and sharing their stories.

But then, in November 2016, our nation elected Donald Trump to the office of President of the United States. I wasn't surprised, not really.

But the book with the witty title now seemed pointless. So I put it away.

Predator-in-Chief

Many first daughters have passed through the White House since I've been old enough to notice. All of them have been sexualized, sexually harassed, and attacked because of their gender.

In 1993, Chelsea Clinton moved in. Her teen awkwardness made her body a target of the political Right: Rush Limbaugh called her a "dog" when she was only thirteen years old.

Then, in 2001, came the Bush twins, Barbara and Jenna. Gorgeous and poised, they were nineteen years old when their father was elected. Even they, the Republican darlings, weren't immune to the sexualization of First Daughter bodies: when they were twenty-three years old, the magazine *Maxim* photoshopped their faces onto the bodies of nearly-naked models having a sexy pillow fight.

Then, in 2009, came Malia and Sasha Obama, the first Black First Daughters, who received the most virulent attacks of all because of their race. For centuries, Black women have been hypersexualized by white people—and white laws—to excuse racist and sexist abuse, from rape by slave owners to rape and abuse that persists today. Thus, the attacks on the Obama daughters were disgusting, but not unexpected.

One notable attack on the Obama daughters came from former Republican congressional aide Elizabeth Lauten, who mocked them on social media: "Dress like you deserve respect, not a spot at a bar." The girls were only thirteen and sixteen years old.

Since 2017, we have had the seemingly cryptic Ivanka

Trump. Age thirty-five when her father Donald Trump was elected, she has served as his stand-in First Lady as well as his political surrogate, especially for white female voters who have a hard time relating to him but see her as evidence that he can't be that bad.

He can't possibly be the sexual predator he seems with a daughter like her.

The Trump family and the Obama family couldn't be more different from one another. Donald Trump is on his third marriage; the Obamas have been married to each other for nearly three decades, since 1992. The Obamas made an especially strong family model in light of the U.S. history of slavery and the institution's deliberate attacks on Black families—and the attacks on Black families that persist to this day.

Yet the public attacks on the sexuality of Michelle Obama and the Obama daughters were relentless—and deeply racist—especially when compared to the lack of such attacks on the Trumps. Donald Trump's third and current wife Melania Trump—who worked as a model and has posed nude in magazines—has caught little flack from the political Right for her work. Nor should she—her career is her own. But condemning women for existing as sexual beings is what the political Right does. They would condemn her roundly if she weren't the wife of a Republican president.

And Donald Trump himself, with his multifarious marriages, his proven record of infidelity and even worse transgressions against women, still manages to maintain the façade of a family man in the eyes of political allies.

In 2016, when Trump was elected president, a certain

message was sent to women in the United States—was sent to me, the would-be author of a book on sexual violence. The message was this: A sexual predator whom we knew preyed on women and girls had been deemed fit for the presidency by the nation we call home. After all, before Trump was elected, we had it all on tape: Trump talking about grabbing pussy, about dating pre-teen girls, about sexualizing his own daughter. Multiple women had credibly accused him of sexual assault—too many to be ignored.

But none of these facts mattered.

Putting Trump into the office of the President of the United States told the men and women of this country, *You can abuse, assault, and demean those who are less powerful than you, and you will not only get away with it, but be rewarded for it.*

Why Now?

I decided to finish this book when the story about Jeffrey Epstein trafficking girls and young women came to light in 2018. But in order to tell you about how the Epstein story affected this book, I need to step back and tell you another story, first.

I've always been afraid of the number 13. There's a name for my fear, triskaidekaphobia, "extreme superstition regarding the number thirteen." Extreme. Don't I know it.

Due to my extreme superstition, I love old-fashioned hotels that skip over thirteen when numbering their floors. I refuse to sit in row thirteen on an airplane. I can't stand writing the date when the date contains the number thirteen.

But: I can never forget that the number thirteen has done me one massive favor in my life. With this book, with its essays on #MeToo and sexual assault, I finally decided to tell the story of that favor. I've been keeping the story a secret for a long, long time.

These days, #MeToo isn't in the news so much—Harvey Weinstein lost his company in 2017. He was arrested in 2018, the same year a jury convicted Bill Cosby. Perhaps all of the giants whom #MeToo could bring down have been brought down. Perhaps.

And once the big names stopped hitting the headlines, the news cycle, unfortunately, moved on.

But there's different news, now. Now, there is Jeffrey Epstein, and the young women he trafficked and sold and raped. In the face of Epstein's arrest and death, in the face of the public testimony by his victims, something changed for me. Because even with all of the essays on sexual assault that I've written and published over the years, there's still one story that I haven't told. But with Epstein's ugly face everywhere, I need to tell it, now.

The Epstein story is so entangled in everything around us: in money, and politics, and men, and power. But in the end, all of that money and power comes down to the exploitation of vulnerable girls and women.

And when I think of that exploitation, I can't help but think of the very ordinary exploitation of one particular, vulnerable girl. And I think that I should tell that story, now. I think that it's time to stop avoiding the story, to stop being afraid to tell it. To realize that I have been afraid.

There are so many who can't tell their stories like mine, but I'm a person who can tell her story. I know that it will hurt me to tell my story, like it always does to tell stories like the ones in this book. It hurts the day I write a story because it hurts to remember. It hurts the day I publish it, when others read it and share their feelings with me. Even when they share their good feelings about what I wrote and their support. Even when they share their mutual sadness. Even when they're not doubting me or accusing me of being an attention whore. It always hurts.

Therefore, before I write a thing that I know will hurt, I don't ask, *Will this hurt?* That's the wrong question, obviously. Of course it will hurt. The right question is: *Is the pain worth the good?* I look at the scales, the good I'm aiming for on one side, and the pain I'll suffer on the other: *Do they sit in balance?*

The chapter "Who's Kay," the reason this book even happened at all, is one I started writing precisely twenty-one years ago. I remember vividly when I started, and when I stopped. I wrote the first draft in graduate school; I was twenty-two years old. When the man across from me in my seminar looked me in the eye and said, "It just doesn't seem that bad," I put the words away and never pulled them out again.

I'm pulling them out now. "Who's Kay" can help answer the questions that so many people ask about young, vulnerable women who are abused by men like Epstein. I know the questions they ask. That man in my graduate seminar said them to me. I say them to myself:

Why did she stay?
Why didn't she leave?
She seemed to like it there with him.
She seemed to like him, period.
She could have run. Why didn't she run?
Why didn't she pick up the phone?
It wasn't like the door was locked.
Why didn't she run out into the street and scream?
Why didn't she scream?

I know all of the answers. They've been locked inside of me for precisely thirty years.

"Who's Kay" took twenty-one years to write because I didn't want to answer those questions. I still don't. The answers will make people feel uncomfortable, even people who believe survivors of rape and abuse. People tend to like clean lines, places to stand firm. The lines in "Who's Kay" are not neat and clean. They're ugly.

I've never written that before, actually. *Ugly*. It feels good to say it. I've kept my story hidden for decades because it is ugly. But I'm old, and I don't care anymore about the ugly. I only wish I'd stopped caring sooner.

I know that if certain people read my ugly story that I will be judged the way all rape survivors are judged. But I will be judged, also, the way survivors who don't scream or fight are judged. The way the ones who stay are judged. This judgment has a particularly sharp edge.

The only thing I have going for me, the only thing I have on my side to protect me from this judgment, the only testimony I can offer, is a number.

Thirteen. I was thirteen.

Overview

Now, near the end of 2019, this book is finally finished, and published, sans witty title.

The book is composed of three parts.

Part One, "The Personal," contains stories about my experiences with sexual harassment and assault and how those experiences have altered other aspects of my life.

Part Two, "The Public," contains stories about how sexual harassment and assault affect our society—legally, institutionally, and so on.

Part Three, "On Campus," focuses on sexual assault on university campuses, on the harassment of students by professors, on the debates around Title IX and other campus laws.

Although some of these chapters were previously published as essays in magazines, they have been heavily revised and expanded for this book. Online writing is a wonderful gift, but its major limitation is the necessity for brevity. Here, I have taken my earlier ideas much further, to the places I never could before.

Most importantly, the chapters in this book provide only a narrow picture of what it means to be a survivor. I'm a white woman in a heterosexual marriage. Although I am disabled—I have bipolar disorder and I am autistic—I have excellent medical care, and I also have the means and access to get my voice heard in national publications and books. I'm not a sex worker or undocumented immigrant or member of any other group who, by the nature of my very identity, is blamed or otherwise further harmed by those who are supposed to help me when I am raped, sexually harassed, or assaulted. Thus: the full picture of rape and sexual assault extends far beyond the pages of this book.

PART I. THE PERSONAL

1

WHY BIRDS HAVE WINGS

She is out with her brother, her brother who knows her. And her brother's Friend who knows her, too. They are all friends. She drinks and she likes to drink. She is good at drinking and not seeming to be drunk especially around her brother, who doesn't like it when she drinks. Her brother's Friend is nice, has always been nice to her, and he's handsome, and a doctor. Her mother would like it if she married a doctor, she thinks, while they sit together in the tall chairs at the bar, drinking. They listen to the music and watch the people dancing. She likes to dance but knows she is too drunk to dance now, she wouldn't dance well, so she sits instead, and listens to the Friend talk about the work he does, about saving people. He is a saver, she thinks: a saver, safe.

It's getting late. The lights are brighter now inside and it is very dark, outside. This means it will be time to go soon. The Friend stands up, steps close to her seat, leans near her, tells her things, tells her that she is beautiful. Beautiful, she thinks, to a man who can have many beautiful things. He puts his hands on her shoulders and squeezes. Her muscles shift shape to fit the shape of his hands, the hands that save people.

They are outside the bar now. Like magic. She doesn't remember how they got there—she and her brother and the Friend. On the sidewalk that tilts toward the street like toward a rushing river. She holds the arm of the Friend and he supports her. She can't stand on her own, she's so drunk, but she pretends she wants to hold on to him, for the pleasure. She smiles at her brother. She reassures her brother. Her brother loves her, she knows. So she smiles and reassures him and tells him she's fine and he believes her. Of course he believes her. She could convince anyone, for a moment on a sidewalk. She convinces her brother that she wants to spend the night at the Friend's house. She trusts the Friend. Her brother trusts him. Why shouldn't she. He is a Friend. A saver. With good hands, magic hands.

It is a sliver of a moment until they arrive at his apartment. Until he is shaking her shoulder telling her to wake because they have arrived. When she wakes, she speaks but she can't speak. Her voice has been stolen and replaced by garbled words that aren't hers. She thinks these words are funny, and laughs as the Friend lifts her from the car. He tells her to be quiet. She tries to say she is sorry, so sorry, but the words fly away like birds.

He carries her inside, dragging her feet across the cement sidewalk, over the metal rim of the sliding glass door. When she feels the carpet under her feet, she considers falling down there and sleeping, knowing the softness will feel like goodness, and she can sleep there. She tries to ask the Friend if she can sleep on the carpet, but he tells her to be quiet, quiet, because his brother is sleeping. The Friend's voice is sharper now, like the rattling of a cage. She stops laughing.

He helps her up the stairs to his room. She sees his bed. She is delighted and falls onto it, lying on her side, pulling her knees to her belly, shutting her eyes, dreaming of sleeping. The Friend disappears into the bathroom. She wonders if he will come back but doesn't care. She is so sleepy and only cares about sleep.

Then he is back and he is on her and he kisses her. She kisses him. She understands kissing. Kissing is nice. He lies on top of her. She can't move her arms because her arms are like her words, no longer hers, garbled, uncontrolled. He pulls her up, holds her with one hand, one fist gripped around her arm, and with the other pulls off her shirt in one motion, then pulls her bra without unclipping it. The tightness of the bra catches on her arms and shoulders but the Friend keeps pulling until it is off of her, until it is gone. He drops her back onto the bed and she falls, falls, until the bed catches her. Now, she cannot shut her eyes, sleep has slipped from her like everything. He stands and removes his shirt, his pants, his everything. He pulls at her pants until the button slips loose, then yanks them from her feet. Her legs are garbled. He reaches for her panties. Her brain turns red. Red red red. She knows, despite this draining, what to do, to say. Magic. Magic words. She moves her muddled arms her mangled fingers to her hips, grabs hold to the edges of her panties, hangs on when the Friend would pull. No, she says. No. No. The only word she knows. The magic word. She holds on and speaks one word.

The Friend grabs her shoulder, squeezes, and turns her over, presses her stomach and face into the blanket, the hard mattress. She doesn't let go of her panties. The Friend slips a finger under the lace edge of her panties between her legs and pulls aside the slender piece of fabric, pulls it aside the distance of two fingers or perhaps the distance of an ocean, and shoves himself inside.

She dies then.

She wakes three hours later to the chirping of birds.

She thinks of her brother first, as she slips out of the Friend's apartment into bright light.

She tells no one. Because she no longer believes in the magic of words.

2

WHY I DIDN'T REPORT BEING RAPED

Here's how it started.
I was raped in grad school and didn't tell anyone. (That's a common story.)

Later, I told someone about my rape, but I didn't report my rape because reporting rape on campus was, and still is, kind of a nightmare. (That's also a common story.)

Later still, I wrote a short story about being raped and published that, but the story was fiction and not real. (It was not real.)

And then, years later, I began doing anti-rape activist work, and the Title IX complaints started happening. I decided to report my rape to the school, hoping that reporting would be less of a nightmare now. (Maybe it was less of a nightmare. But it was still a nightmare.)

But.

I never reported my rape to the police—even though, even now, I could. North Carolina, the state where I live, where he raped me, has no statute of limitations for felonies.

No statute of limitations. What he did will always be a crime. In my eyes, and in the eyes of the law. Right?

Sort of.

That's the problem.

Why didn't you report being raped?

Other people ask me that question, sure. But mostly I ask myself.

Why didn't I report being raped?—I ask myself that question a lot. And then I torture myself with the answers.

Why didn't you report being raped?

Because my rapist is a doctor and no one will believe that a doctor would do something like that.

Because I was basically cheating on my boyfriend when I went home with my rapist. And even though I didn't want to have sex with my rapist, that won't matter in the eyes of a prosecutor or jury.

Because I have a psychiatric disability that will torpedo my credibility in the eyes of anyone, and I mean anyone, who knows anything about prosecuting rape or defending against rape charges. I am a lawyer, and I know that anyone with a psychiatric disability like mine would have her credibility as a witness destroyed by even the most poorly trained, overworked, and nervous defense attorney.

Because I know that my psychiatric disability will come out in court, no matter what the rules of evidence say. It will. And I will have to listen to them, the members of the self-same profession that I'm a part of, doing defense work that I know is important, I will have to listen to them destroy my credibility as a witness to my own rape on the basis of a psychiatric disability that has absolutely nothing to do with my credibility as a witness in the world of empirical fact, but everything to do with my credibility as a witness in the world of stigma and bigotry.

Because I don't know if I will survive that experience.

Why didn't you report being raped?

Because I was so drunk on the drinks my rapist gave me at the bar that I passed out in my rapist's car while he drove me to his apartment and so I didn't even know where we were. My drunken state didn't matter much to me until after he raped me. After he raped me, I didn't know how to get home. So I asked him to drive me. And then later I realized that asking him to drive me home would give a defense attorney even more ammo against me because why would I ask him to drive me home if I was afraid of him? Why would I choose to spend more time with him if he was a rapist? Why didn't I just run out of his apartment and start screaming? Isn't that how a rape victim is supposed to act?

Because I didn't act how a rape victim is supposed to act.

Because I couldn't remember which of the little towns his apartment was located in. When I think about reporting to the police, I realize that I don't even know which police station to report my rape to because I don't know which police force has jurisdiction over my rape.

Because I don't want to even think about the word jurisdiction.

Because after I was raped, I hated myself and wanted to die. And I still kind of do, even years and years later.

Why didn't you report being raped?

Because my rapist was a friend of my family, and I didn't know if they would take his side.

Because I knew that if my family took my rapist's side I wouldn't have a family anymore. So I thought it would be better not to put the issue to the test.

Because the first time I was raped, when I was a child, adults blamed me for it. My animal brain is still really confused about that. My animal brain knows that being blamed hurts and believes that keeping secrets is less painful than risking being blamed again.

Because I can't believe that I am a person who was raped twice. What does it say about me that I am a person who was raped twice? Am I a perpetual victim? Am I doomed to be victimized, attacked, forever?

Because maybe my brain really is broken. Because maybe it really is my fault, if it happened to me twice.

Right?

3

BEING COUNTED

REPORTING MY RAPE AT A SCHOOL UNDER TITLE IX INVESTIGATION

The first thing I have to do is find out X.'s full name. I know his first and last name, but I want to have his middle name. Being able to say all three names has power. Like when I get mad at my kids and say all three names, they know they're in deep shit.

I don't even know how to spell X.'s first name properly —it's a name with a couple of possible spellings. Since I figure he'll be a practicing doctor now, I just Google him. I don't think twice. I type his name into the search bar and Google takes me right to his home page. To the page of his plastic surgery practice in one of the wealthiest towns in the United States.

Cheesy synth-jazz plays in the background while I stare into the eyes of my rapist.

I am not prepared for this.

I am not prepared to look into his eyes after so many years. After one doctorate, one marriage, and two children. This is not something I could ever have been prepared for. I hit mute on my computer.

I hate this man. I hate that he has a plastic surgery practice. The menu for the work he does divides women into body parts like "thighs," "face," "breasts," and "torso." Women's eyes stare at me through my screen. His homepage looks like a fucking porno site. I get his full name and shut the browser.

I type his name into the rape reporting notes that I'm preparing to bring with me to campus. The notes feel inauthentic when compared to the report of, say, an undergraduate in a moment of crisis. But I know I will fight similar battles to the young women reporting rapes after finding themselves naked in frat house broom closets or basements.

The rape reporting people on campus will want details (details I won't have). They will want to tell me what to do with my report, perhaps take it to the police (and I will have to resist them because for many reasons I can't deal with the police). They will quickly form ideas about what kind of person I am the minute I walk through the door (and those ideas will likely be wrong).

Because they will want details, I'm preparing notes. My first problem is that I don't remember the date. Fortunately, I'm detail-obsessed. I've kept journals since age thirteen to record everything. So that's the first place I look to find the date. But, for some reason, I didn't write down much about X. raping me. I didn't write down the date. This is very unlike me. (Note to Past Me: What were you thinking?)

No problem, though, because I also keep a detailed calendar. Like, if Adrian Monk decided to keep a calendar, he would be jealous of my calendar. He'd ask me for calendar lessons. I start flipping through my past calendars, year by year, to the calendar for 20– ... and it is gone. Fucking gone. They're all lined up on the shelf, and that one is missing.

Now, I wouldn't have written in the calendar "Raped by X." on whatever day in 20–. But I would have written down when I was flying to visit a guy that I'd just started dating. The reason I was in Chapel Hill at all, instead of in Greensboro where I was attending graduate school, was to stay overnight with my sister so I could fly out of the Raleigh airport the next morning on Southwest Airlines.

In the early morning hours before that flight, X. raped me.

I still caught that flight. No, I didn't tell the guy I was dating that I was raped. How would that have gone? "Hey Y.! Great to see you! I know this relationship is brand new and that it's long-distance anyways so things are delicate but guess what! This guy I was having drinks with and got kissy with last night raped the shit out of me at his apartment! Wanna talk about it?"

Um, no.

I keep thinking of X.'s smug-ass face on his creepy-ass synth-jazz website. His website needs a trigger warning for anyone with taste.

I start searching my hard drive for flight confirmations from Southwest Airlines for this 20– trip. I find it. The flight departed on July 27, which means I was raped around three o'clock in the morning on July 27, 20–.

Can this be it? The day? I imagined that I would feel something when I encountered the date.

I feel nothing.

I don't believe the date is right. I have to be sure. Maybe

I flew up twice out of Raleigh. But I can't find any other saved tickets on my hard drive.

I call the airline. This takes forever. I can't get through to anyone who has information. The last person I speak to on the phone tells me data that old has been "archived."

I email my old boyfriend Y. For a minute, I can't believe I'm doing this. I don't tell him why. I just say that I need the dates that I came to visit him. He tells me that he doesn't have those old emails anymore. (Hi Y.! This is why I emailed you about those dates, by the way.)

Emails! I go into Gmail. (Google: Thanks for not being evil and for saving my old emails.) I keyword search by the airport call letters where Y. lives, and it pulls up a second itinerary on Southwest. There it is. That's the day. I can feel it.

It was in August. I know it was in August. Believe me if you've ever lived in North Carolina then you know when something happened in August.

August 23, 20–. My day.

I have to write the narrative of what happened that night to give to UNC. As I write it, I think about the genre of the rape narrative. This is a document that so many women have to write. We should gather these horrible documents together and publish them, these tortured little stories that must comply with the parameters of procedure.

I decide to push the genre boundaries a little bit. That is my professorial specialty: genre theory. How the use and reuse of language takes shape in the form of predictable texts. I'm already unpredictable: a professor reporting to her college.

I wonder how much I care about what these people are

going to think of me. I'm not sure I know the answer. What has started out as a clinical exercise has stopped feeling so clinical.

Next step: How does a person who's been raped report a rape at UNC these days? Back to Google!

I type, "report rape UNC."

The first hit reads like this: "College student could be expelled for reporting her rape…," a New York Daily News story on a UNC student apparently facing expulsion for reporting her rapist.[1]

The second hit takes me to SAFE@UNC, which seems to be the right place for reporting a rape.

(The next four hits are also about UNC students getting in trouble for reporting rape. UNC needs some SEO help.)

The SAFE@UNC website has major design flaws. But the "get help" link is right next to the webpage name, so I click it.

This "get help" page is even worse than the home page. At the top are three bullet points telling you what to do in an emergency: "Call 911" is first, followed by calling campus police, and then going to the hospital emergency department. These are fine instructions, though not helpful to me. I read on.

The three bullet points are followed by a page of text so dense it looks like it was written by Don DeLillo.

I read it all. There are no subheadings, just random phrases in boldface. Under the paragraph that tells me, "The University can provide help and support," the first person named has this title: "Deputy Title IX/Student Complaint Coordinator." I don't understand what it means to coordinate Title IX in a deputy fashion, but I do know that I want to file a complaint.

OK, I think. I'll try him. (And yes, he's a man.) I get his voicemail. His recording says to call 911 if there is an emergency, otherwise to leave a message.

I don't leave a message.

The second person named in the DeLillean paragraph has this title: "Title IX Coordinator." I'm guessing he's the boss, since the first guy is only a deputy. I call the second guy. (Yes, also a man.)

This time a woman answers the phone. From the tone of her voice, it seems she answers phones for a living.

"Hello! Equal opportunity!"

I'm not sure I have the right place, since she didn't say anything about Title IX, but I forge ahead.

"I need to report a rape," I say. Also, I realize now that my heart is racing.

The woman has no idea what to say to me. I've totally thrown her off. After a few moments, she articulates that she needs to figure out who to transfer me to. She puts me on hold with really fucking loud marching band music. It's like the music you would hear at half-time at a football game. I'm glad I wasn't raped by a football player or a member of the marching band.

If it had been synth-jazz, I would have lost my bananas.

She comes back and tells me she's going to transfer me to a person named Camille. I don't know who this Camille person is, but I don't ask, because the secretary seems so flustered. She's having such a hard time figuring out what to do with someone who wants to report a rape.

Camille, conversely, has her stuff together.

"I want to report a rape," I say, and Camille doesn't hesitate. She asks me to tell her more about myself. I tell her I'm a current UNC professor, but that the rape happened a few years ago when I was a graduate student.

At that point, Camille tells me I'm in the wrong place. "I hate to transfer you," she says. Because X. and I were students at the time of the rape, my case has to be handled by the Title IX office. I tell her that only my rapist was a UNC student—I was a UNCG student. She tells me that doesn't matter, the Title IX office handles the case.

She takes my name and number, and tells me that she'll have someone from the Title IX office call me. Then she asks me, as though she still can't quite believe it, "And you're a professor here?"

"Yes." I say. I feel an iota of joy. This is the only power I have in this entire affair.

I tell her, just before we hang up, that it was the Title IX office who transferred me to her in the first place.

She sounds exasperated and tells me that she'll just take the "details" herself.

I say okay, and then I ask, "What details?"

She means she wants to take my report over the phone.

I say, "Can I come in person to report?" She says nothing. I say, quickly, "I have the whole day free. I can come this afternoon."

She says she'll call me back to set up a time. I ask if she has my phone number. She reads it back to me, and she's written it down incorrectly. I give her my correct number, we hang up, and I wait.

I hate waiting.

About twenty minutes and one plate of microwave

nachos later, the phone rings, and it's Camille again. She says she's calling to make sure that someone from the Title IX office got in touch with me. I tell her no one has called. She tells me that she spoke with "Howie" directly, and so I should be hearing from someone soon.

I say, "Howie?"

And then I realize she's talking about Howard, the Title IX Coordinator. She tells me he's "in charge over there." I'm still not clear about where these different offices are located, and why there are multiple offices in the first place. But I just say thank you, and we hang up.

I ask myself, if it were back in 20– right after I was raped, at what point in this process would I have lost my cool and given up reporting this rape at all?

Somewhere around the nachos.

I want to report a rape. How do those words not create a DEFCON 1 situation in our rape reporting office?

I don't know. I'm just eating nachos and waiting for a phone call.

I called at 10:50 a.m. Camille called me back at 11:20 a.m.

At 2:15 that afternoon, the Deputy Title IX/Student Complaint Coordinator finally calls me, the person directly under "Howie."

When you are waiting to report a rape, with your neatly typed rape narrative frying a hole in your purse, waiting three and a half hours to finally talk to someone is more like waiting three and a half years. I can't concentrate on anything. My heart won't slow down.

I didn't know it would be like this after so long.

On the phone, the man tells me that he's leaving town tomorrow and the soonest he can meet with me is the end of next week. Or, he tells me, I can meet with one of his associates in his office sooner than that, and he'll follow up with me for more details. My head spins with all of these meetings I'm supposed to have and the fact that I have to wait so long to have them.

I tell him that I've set aside today, Tuesday, to report my rape, so I would like to meet with someone this afternoon. "That's why I called this morning to make an appointment," I say. I realize I'm panicking a little.

He seems taken aback by my request, but quickly recovers.

He tells me where his office is located. It's actually off of campus in an office building that I've never heard of even though I've more or less lived in the area for twenty years.

"Where should I park?" I ask.

He says they don't have reserved parking spaces, but I can parallel park on Franklin Street—the busy thoroughfare through town. He says, unfortunately, that his office can't validate the parking fees.

He asks me how long it will take me to get to his office. I tell him five minutes. I'm relieved that he seems game to meet with me so quickly.

Thumbs up.

On my way down Franklin Street, I pass the bar where X. and I were hanging out the evening before he raped me. It's still there, on the same street as the place where I'm going to report being raped.

After I find parking, I enter the double glass doors of the building where his directions tell me to go. I get on the elevator and head to the top floor. I step off and find myself in a long hallway like any long hallway in an office building. I can't believe I've never seen this place before.

I head into the office suite. There's a woman entering in front of me. She asks me who I'm there to see. "E.W." I say, pronouncing his name the way he said it to me on the phone. E.W., the Deputy Title IX/Student Complaint Coordinator.

The woman steps into an office and tells someone I'm there.

He comes out to greet me. He's a white man as tall as I am, maybe taller, and has blond hair and fair skin. We shake hands. He invites me into his office. One wall is composed of windows looking into the office suite. They're covered in open mini-blinds.

We sit at a round laminate table. The office furniture is brand new. The outlets on the baseboards don't have outlet covers on them yet.

He first tells me it is part of his job to take in complaints like mine, but he assures me that the word "complaints" is a "policy term." He seems worried I might get hung up on it. But I don't know if he thinks I'll take the word too seriously, or not seriously enough.

Then he says that everything I share with him will be "private" but not "confidential." I ask him to explain. He says that he shares information with his team, gesturing through the glass windows at the other people in the office. He's also required to report rapes to the UNC Department of Public Safety, but he doesn't give victims' names unless victims want him to. He says that DPS keeps track of the numbers of rapes for Clery Act purposes.[2]

I feel defeated. I know that universities must keep Clery

Act logs of all crimes reported to them for seven years. If the UNC DPS only keeps logs for the maximum amount of time the Act requires, then my rape will not be logged at all.

But he's sitting in front of me with a very official-looking form. Something official is happening here in this Title IX office. He, and his form, reassure me that what I'm doing isn't for nothing.

I have my typed-up report on the table in front of me. I'm hesitating to hand it over. I realize why.

"Honestly, I'm scared of libel," I tell him. I'm afraid X. will somehow find out about the report and come after me because of what is in it. I think about those search results on Google for "report rape UNC."

I tell him I don't want to pursue any legal action against X. Even though North Carolina has no statute of limitations for felonies, I tell him, laughing, that I know no prosecutor would take my case. I also don't want to pursue University action. (I don't even know if University action still exists.) I don't want to do anything but report being raped and have it recorded.

It seems important to tell him these things before I hand him my report. I want him to understand I don't have any motive for acting against X. other than having my rape counted. I'm not trying to bring the good doctor down. I'm not a vindictive bitch who is having "regrets" after having "one too many."

I can't believe I'm even thinking these things.

I hand him the report.

"Do you mind if I read this through?" he asks.

I shake my head.

He reads it. While he's reading, I feel nervous and exposed. I feel my body in strange ways. I stare at the outlets with no outlet covers.

He finishes reading the report. He asks, "This website is his current business?"

"Yes."

"Do you remember the location of his apartment?"

"Nope."

He asks me if there's anything else I'd like to add to the report. I don't understand the question and ask if his question is meant to imply something else. He says no, that sometimes people want to add things when they talk. I say no, everything is typed in the report.

He asks me, "Why now?"

I try to figure out what he wants to know. Does he want to know why, after all of these years, I want to report at all? Does he want to know if something changed in my life? Does he want to know why this year instead of last year, or today instead of yesterday?

I do my best to explain. I start by telling him why I didn't report at the time I was raped. I didn't report because I was flying out a few hours after being raped to visit my sort-of-long-distance-boyfriend-person. I just wanted to pretend being raped didn't happen and focus on the other guy.

(To that Southwest Airlines flight attendant who brought me the three gigantic plastic trash bags to fill with vomit during that flight and gave me my own row to sit in and then brought me fifteen cans of ginger ale, and the whole time made jokes to cheer me up while you hauled away my mess: Bless you. I hope you are a Gordon-Gekko-level boss now.)

I didn't report at the time because I was a lawyer. (A young, newbie lawyer, but still a lawyer.) Because I was a lawyer, while I was vomiting into trash bags on that plane, I coldly assessed the merits of my case. If you were a prosecutor, would you take on your case? No.

I didn't report at the time because I knew that rape reports that didn't get prosecuted ended up in the hinterlands of this-makes-the-school-look-bad-let's-ignore-it.

(Plus, you know, I hated myself and wanted to die.)

I tell him that since the Title IX office has started informing the UNC faculty (that means me) about the new Title IX office and their fiercer rules about information-gathering—no more hinterlands or burying of complaints—it seems like a good time to say something. So that's why now.

He asks me, "Are you okay?"

"I'm okay," I say. I feel tears rush to my eyes. I force them back. Then I wonder if it would be better to just cry. Would that make me seem more genuine? I mean, I am genuine. But do I seem too cold because I'm not crying? Does he expect victims to cry? But if I cry, will I seem less believable because I'm too emotional?

I don't cry.

He tells me about counseling services, the rape crisis center, the women's center, and the woman who runs the crisis unit at Chapel Hill P.D. He asks if my husband is supportive.

In short, he was great, once I was finally able to get over

the hurdles that (1) I had to wait for hours (2) to speak to a dude about being raped (3) in a strange off-campus building with no parking. He even listened to me when I told him how unfortunate the SAFE@UNC website is. (He inherited it. They're working on it right now.)

Before I leave, I warn him about the creepy synth-jazz. I tell him to prepare himself, because that shit is terrible.

4

OVER NOTHING

Three times this week.

Three times this week, a loud noise or a trick of light convinced me that something terrible was about to happen to the people whom I love most: my husband, my two sons.

Three times this week, a misperception caused my brain, nervous system, body to have an overwhelming, involuntary reaction.

You could call these reactions panic attacks, and you might be right—my doctor isn't quite sure. But, she is sure that they are a post-traumatic stress reaction of some sort.

Here's what happens: I am suddenly unable to breathe; my heart races and feels as though it is going to break through my ribs; I cannot see very well; I feel fear-driven confusion. The reaction can last for thirty seconds or thirty minutes.

After the reaction ends, I feel sucked dry of energy, and also emotion. I feel a strange need to cry—but I try to avoid crying—exhausted, emotional tears. My hands and arms shiver and shake. It takes an hour or so before my body is back to normal.

Sometimes, though, the reaction happens in the middle of the night—in that case, there is no back to normal. I cannot go back to sleep. I give up on getting any rest and stare out the window, impatient for the sun to rise.

The third reaction this week happened at 5:30 in the morning, as my husband drove me to the airport with our two children in the back seat of the car. It was so early that the sun had yet to rise. Suddenly, I saw a deer about to dash into the road, in front of our car, and I screamed.

But no. There was no deer. What I saw was a trick caused by a streetlight shining through a spindly tree, casting long shadows on the side of the road. My husband, accustomed to my fearful outbursts, rested his hand on my knee to reassure me that all was well. As my heart slowed again, I worked hard not to cry in front of the kids.

After a few minutes, my five-year-old asked me, "Mommy, why are you always screaming over nothing?"

Then he and his seven-year-old brother laughed at the hilarious joke.

I was so happy to hear them laughing.

"I have no idea," I said, laughing with them. I wanted their memory of my departure to be one of joy.

My husband squeezed my hand.

———

I HAVE panic reactions because I was raped. Sometimes they happen in public: when I'm doing events related to rape, like giving talks or readings. Sometimes they happen in private: when I'm doing work about rape, like watching movies about rape or writing pieces about rape. Sometimes they happen for no reason related to rape at all, because of a loud noise or a trick of light. The worst part is how unpredictable these panic reactions are. They happen in the grocery store. They happen at my sister's house. They happen around my kids.

It is impossible to know whether I would have developed these reactions after being raped if I did not also have a psychiatric disability. A major study of post-traumatic stress disorder (PTSD) in rape victims specifically excluded victims who had pre-existing mental health conditions. For reference, the 1992 study (by Rothbaum et al. in the *Journal of Traumatic Stress*) found that, after three months, 47% of rape victims suffered from PTSD. Furthermore, if you are a rape victim suffering from PTSD after the three month mark, you are far less likely to recover over time.

By contrast, the Department of Veterans Affairs reports that PTSD rates from the Vietnam era to today in active-duty combat military personnel range from 20-30% at the highest.

Being raped is traumatic. It's a war over your body, even. It's more traumatic than most people might have imagined, until you tell them the numbers.

But I don't only have PTSD. I have a psychiatric disability. For example, I have anxiety disorder, which makes everything harder, including PTSD.

Indeed, the two—severe trauma and psychiatric disability—make for a tough combination for everyone.

And although people like me were excluded by Rothbaum et al., what the Rothbaum study showed us for sure is that you do not have to have a psychiatric disability to develop PTSD after being raped. Nearly half of all rape victims do.

You don't have to have a disability to end up "a mess," after.

But having a psychiatric disability does make rape victims more vulnerable to developing PTSD after being raped. And, having a disability, including a psychiatric disability, according to the National Crime Victimization Survey, makes you more vulnerable to being raped in the first place.

I was vulnerable, very vulnerable, because of my disability.

Now that I am older—now that I am a rape victim—I am far more careful with how I drink alcohol. Now I know that one drink—just one—can make me drunk. Or, I can have three and not be the slightest bit tipsy. What I know for certain is that I can never predict what my body's reaction will be because I can never predict how my body will have metabolized my psychiatric medication throughout the day.

But, when I was younger, still learning how the medicines worked with my body, and when I was still more trusting of those around me, I was less careful with alcohol. Less, you might say, paranoid.

So, when I tell you that I was drunk the night that I was raped in graduate school, drunk after drinking at a bar with other students whom I trusted, you might imagine a typical night out, with a group of friends throwing back drinks, a girl who should have been more careful (paranoid). But nothing about having a severe psychiatric disability is typical.

It changes everything.

I did not consent.

I did say "no" (over and over). My rapist held me down with his elbow across the back of my neck.

What I have learned about the interaction of psychiatric disability and rape is this: I cannot separate the before (I am disabled), from the event (I am a disabled person who was raped), from the aftermath (I am a person who was raped, who then developed a disability called PTSD).

AND THEN THERE is the rest of the aftermath.

At the time I was raped, I did not report my rape to the police because I knew that I would not be believed. I knew that I would not be believed not (only) because I had been drinking, but also because I have a psychiatric disability. People with psychiatric disabilities are deemed, by our very nature, to be untrustworthy witnesses to our own lives.

Don't believe a thing she says. She's crazy.

But, I'm not an outlier. Most rape victims do not report being raped. There are lots of reasons to avoid reporting. If you are raped at college, as we all now know (and as I write about later in this book), universities do a notoriously bad job helping rape victims who report being raped. Organizations like End Rape on Campus (EROC) and *The*

Hunting Ground film have shined some light on this problem.

But universities also do a bad job handling the ways that disability and rape often unfold together.

For example: A student is raped. After being raped, she develops PTSD, which is—what studies show—a normal reaction. She grows anxious and depressed. Anxiety and depression cause insomnia. Lack of sleep means she has trouble making it to class. Poor class attendance causes her to do poorly in her classes. Her poor performance makes her more depressed. She is also afraid to leave her room for fear of seeing her rapist and his enabling friends around campus. She stops eating. She stops exercising. She grows even more depressed.

Sometimes, as in the case of Lizzy Seeberg, Sasha Menu Courey, and countless other rape victims who have died by suicide, this normal, post-rape traumatic reaction kills her.

Women do not die by suicide after being raped because they are weak. They die by suicide because depression and other post-trauma reactions can be deadly, and institutions do not provide rape victims the support and intervention that they need.

Depression is a psychiatric disability, as is PTSD. And yet when I (finally) reported my rape to my institution, they showed no particular urgency to get me any sort of disability services. It was as though no one on campus knew the incredibly high incidence of psychiatric disability in rape victims. Forty-seven percent after three months is an epidemic.

Or, perhaps the people in those institutions knew, but they didn't care. I'm not sure. Or, perhaps they cared, but the number, the forty-seven percent, is so high, so overwhelming, that they know they could do nothing meaningful to help.

All I know is, ten years later, I am still screaming. But not, despite all the time that has passed, over nothing.

5

EVEN IF YOU'RE BROKEN

I decided to take a train. The distance between Chapel Hill, North Carolina, and Washington, D.C., is too far for me to drive alone without getting antsy and too close to fly without feeling like I'm wasting an immense amount of money. My friends say Megabus is the best way to travel, but trains have their allure: the big seats, the big views, the rumble, the speed—both fast and slow at the same time.

A train it was.

My train was, naturally, late. My train was late because I live below the Mason-Dixon line, and below the Mason-Dixon line the trains are notoriously unreliable. But that was okay. I'd given myself plenty of time to get to D.C. before the event started. I'd given myself time to change into my dress and to mentally prepare to meet lots of new people.

I was heading up for the book launch event at the Sixth & I Historic Synagogue for the book *We Believe You: Survivors of Campus Sexual Assault Speak Out*. I'd contributed a chapter, and the thirty-six contributors had all been invited to come to the launch. Scattered all over the world like we were, we couldn't all make it, but I could.

Writing my chapter for *We Believe You* was not the first time I'd written about the things I wrote about. I'd already written about the story of being raped, about reporting my campus rape years after it happened, about why I didn't report being raped back when it first happened, about trying to take my own life, and about being a mom —all of those things wrapped up in a terrible and beautiful package. *We Believe You* wasn't even the first book I'd been a part of. On the contrary, by the time the book came out, I'd published many books, both nonfiction and novels.

Way back when the two editors of *We Believe You* first asked me to contribute, I was hesitant. I'd already told my "rape story," I thought. Also, as a professional writer, I'm hesitant to write for free, and the contributors to the collection weren't paid. But the editors are dear to me, and I believe in their work, so I agreed. I put my piece together and that was that. I didn't think much more about it.

And then, as the months went by, being a part of *We Believe You* started to matter more. I formed a relationship, via phone and email, with the book's editor at the publishing house. To see how much of her heart she'd thrown into the project made me wonder if perhaps I were missing something.

That feeling—*Am I missing something?*—is not unusual for me. I often underestimate important events.

Because I wondered if I were missing something, I booked a train. And then I was on that train to D.C. for the book launch at the Sixth & I. I put on a dress. I arrived at the venue in a hired car with the book's editors along with another contributor, named A.

Another friend had gone ahead to Sixth & I to arrange things, kind of like an advance guard. When our car arrived at the venue, the advance guard shuttled us in the back door. "It's crazy out there," the advance guard told us. "Sneak in this way."

It's crazy out there?

That's when my heart started to beat a little funny. I ignored my body. After all, I'm an author. I've read to crowds. I've given keynote lectures to theaters full of people. This event, I told myself, was not a big deal.

But, like I said, I tend to underestimate things. I was about to be proven very wrong.

The advance guard led us into the green room, where some bookstore ladies had set out copies of *We Believe You* for the two editors to sign. One of the editors asked how many folks were out in the auditorium proper. "Nearly three hundred!" the bookstore lady answered. "Amazing!"

That's when I had my panic attack.

———

PANIC ATTACKS HAPPEN NOW and then. In large crowds, when I'm home alone with my kids late at night, when I'm startled by a loud noise, when I saw the documentary on campus rape *The Hunting Ground* for the first time in a crowded antique theater in Chapel Hill.

About an hour into *The Hunting Ground*, I started to feel shaky. My heart started to race. So I texted my friend who starred in the film to ask how much longer the film would be—should I leave now? Should I try to stick it out? Before I could finish composing the text, this horrible woman seated next to me scolded me for taking out my phone.

"Put your phone away," she hissed. "You're being rude."

I stood, crossing in front of her, and rushed from the theater. Her scolding sent me into the lobby of The Chelsea Theater where, once I was under the bright lights, I leaned against the wall, slid down to the floor, and curled into a ball, sobbing.

One of the teenaged boys selling popcorn came rushing over and asked if he should call 911.

I waited there until my friend arrived, the one who starred in the film. I told her what happened.

Maybe if the woman hadn't scolded me I wouldn't have broken down. Maybe. I don't know. I do know that all future screenings of *The Hunting Ground* included a pre-screening statement telling viewers that they could send text messages if they needed to.

This is what the onset of a post-traumatic panic attack feels like for me: I can only see right in front of me because my peripheral vision seems to fade away. I tend to squeeze whatever I'm holding very hard. If I'm not holding anything, then I squeeze my own hands. I've hurt myself doing this, torn the skin between my fingers, without noticing. I'm unable to answer questions properly, or make decisions. I get very quiet, and back away from everyone. I'm one second away from sobbing on the floor.

AT THAT MOMENT in the green room, the three hundred or more attendees seated just outside, the bookstore ladies told us they didn't have seats in the front reserved for contributors.

Instead, they told us that we'd have to squeeze into the room full of three hundred people, seated alone, sprinkled throughout, finding seats at the last minute.

At the thought of sitting alone among strangers, in an overcrowded room filled with three hundred people, where we were going to spend hours talking about rape, my vision narrowed, my ears started ringing, and I backed up against the wall.

I realized what was happening.

I turned to A., the other contributor who'd ridden in the car with me, and said, "I have to leave now. Right now."

So much for the train ride. For wanting to be there for something that seemed like it might be important. For taking two full days away from my husband and kids just for this one event for this one book.

This is what it means to be a rape survivor. You are surprised, constantly, by your brokenness.

A., the other contributor, called one of the editors over from where she was signing books. A. told her about the seating situation. The editor was annoyed, angry even.

She politely informed the bookstore ladies that the books' contributors needed reserved seating at the front of the venue, and they needed it now. Folding chairs were located and set up in the front of the house. Or so I heard, from A., who, I think, was holding my hand.

And then we were walking out. And then I was sitting with my back to a large room of people, but because they were to my back, I could pretend they weren't there. And then I could watch my friends on stage with a United States senator as the emcee, talking about the book I was a part of, and I could feel so proud of them and of what they had accomplished. And I could stay after and meet the book's other contributors, most of whom I'd only connected with on social media, and realize why the book was, indeed, special.

Because we are the survivors. Despite the ways that we go about our days mostly whole or mostly broken or partly whole or partly broken or sometimes entirely broken, we are still here.

That means something.

So. To the person who has never told anyone but the bathroom mirror that you were raped: I believe you. We believe you. Even if you're broken. Like me.

6

READING ROMANCE WHEN YOU WERE NEVER A VIRGIN

I'm reading my way through a romance series. I'm on the fifth installment, and I've gotten a feel for the unique quirks of the books as well as for the ways the books heed romance novel conventions—especially the less enticing conventions.

The convention I'm having trouble dealing with most, one of the most common romance novel conventions of all, is this: All of the heroines, no matter what their age, no matter what century they were born in (there's some time-traveling involved), are virgins when they meet the heroes.

There's nothing wrong with being a virgin, of course. Lots of people are virgins, even into their mid-twenties (or later), just like the heroines of the novels I'm reading. But lately, the way virginity is used as a trope in romance novels has started to get to me.

Although there are exceptions, it is unusual to read a historical romance novel without encountering a virginal heroine. It's simply that common of a genre convention.

What's the big deal?

The big deal, for me, is the particular trope of virginity-as-sacred-gift to the hero. The big deal, for me, is the other trope of virginity-as-stand-in-for-honesty, resolve, valor, courage, and an assortment of other qualities that a romance heroine has no other way of proving she possesses except by guarding her hymen.

In a romance novel that uses these tropes, when the moment of truth—that is, cherry-picking—finally comes, and inevitably the reader enters the hero's point of view for at least a moment, he feels such gratitude that he's the one to have received the gift of the heroine's virginity. And in that moment, he truly admires her.

And in that moment, I feel sick and cheated. I feel like a failure. I wonder why I'm reading the book and consider stopping. Every time. But I set aside my bad feelings and keep reading. After all, it's not the romance novel genre's fault that I was raped when I was a child and never had a chance to be a virgin at all.

———

WHEN I WAS a freshman in college, my best friend was a girl named Bel. She and I were walking through the student union during what turned out to be rape awareness week. I, of course, was so wildly unaware of everything in college that I didn't know such a week even existed.

A campus activist group had set up a long, white bulletin board—a memorial. It stretched as long as the building itself. When Bel and I found it, the board was covered by a flurry of yellow index cards, so many that the board looked like a field of daffodils. On a nearby table were more cards, along with pens and push-pins so you could write a note and stick it on the board.

I'd never told Bel what happened to me as a child, so I was nervous about writing anything on a card. But she strode to the table, picked up a card and wrote a note, and then stabbed it into the board. Her note read, *For the girl who never got to be a virgin.*

For a moment, I had a strange feeling that Bel had read my mind. She could have written that note about me. She hadn't, though. I quickly wrote a note for myself, and we walked outside onto the quad. We sat in the spring North Carolina sunshine on a patch of grass by the gothic-inspired chapel and told each other very similar stories.

Then, Bel told me she had a theory. It went like this: Since she never had a chance to choose whom to have sex with the first time, she got to be a virgin forever.

Bel was an eternal virgin.

AT FIRST GLANCE, Bel's theory seemed similar to the advice given by nurse practitioner Carol F. Roye, writing in 2014 for the *Our Bodies, Ourselves* website about about the uselessness of our cultural misconceptions about hymens and virginity: "I believe that virginity is what the individual thinks it is. It certainly is for men, who bear no tell-tale signs of lost virginity. The concept of virginity has an emotional connotation. It is more than just the physical disruption of hymenal tissue."

Roye, however, was not advising a perception of virginity until you felt like you weren't a virgin anymore.

On the contrary, she was advising women to take a broader, not narrower, view of virginity loss: "If a young woman has had a sexual relationship with her partner, and she feels that she has lost her virginity, then she has, regardless of what actually happened to her hymen during the encounter. There are ancillary issues that each woman must answer for herself. Is oral sex 'de-virginizing?' Anal sex?"

No: Bel had flipped Roye's advice on its head. Bel had declared herself a virgin for as long as she wanted to be one.

Roye's advice didn't take into consideration me or Bel or other women like us at all. When I read her article I needed an answer to a very specific question: How do you think about virginity when yours was gone before you were a sexual being in the first place?

JUST A FEW MONTHS before my conversation with Bel, I'd had sex for the first time since I was raped by a grown man when I was in middle school.

My first adult sexual experience was not the most romantic experience in the world. In fact, in retrospect, I don't think I wanted it to be. I think I wanted to get it over with. I didn't have a hymen (metaphorical or no) to discard, but I did have plenty of baggage. I chose someone I knew I would never see again—an ex-boyfriend from high school. I selected him carefully for a one-night stand.

In retrospect.

Before we went at it, I told Ex-Boyfriend I was raped

when I was a child—I'd never told him before. He seemed, weirdly, relieved. "So you're not a virgin, then."

What did that question mean? That he was going to do things differently? Would he have done things differently if I'd said nothing? What if I'd had the eternal virgin conversation with Bel sooner and kept my rape a secret from him? What if I'd told him I was a virgin—what would have happened then? Did he think my body was transformed somehow by its less-than-virginal status, and his own duty to me therefore lightened?

Sarah Wendell at the romance novel website *Smart Bitches, Trashy Books* addressed what she called the "Surprise Virgin" trope in romance novels. It goes like this:

> The hero figures out the heroine is a virgin because he encounters some resistance (which, don't even get me started) and she flinches and of course he Is Very Alarmed and tries to stop but she tells him not to so it's ok for him to get on with it. Then after they've crested and reached peaks of joy and done the dance as old as time, he says something about how if he'd known she was a virgin, he'd have done it all differently, been more gentle or something.

Wendell has all kinds of criticisms of this particularly weak trope: "First, why would you not bring your A game the first time you sleep with a woman you have major lust pants for? If your groin is on fire and it's not because of Gold Bond, why would you not do your very best scrumpin? What is this 'I'd have been more gentle and sensitive' crap?"

Ex-Boyfriend and I had the awkward I-was-raped

conversation. Then I, with my non-virginal eighteen-year-old body, and he, with his extremely non-virginal twenty-year-old body, fucked in my friend's guest room. It hurt like hell. I cried and made sure he didn't see. Sex felt terrible, and I never wanted to do it again. Maybe that was his A game. Maybe it wasn't.

My de-baggaging (you really can't call it deflowering) did not involve peaks of joy.

I was an unusual species of surprise virgin. I'd been deflowered, yes, when I was a child. But in no way was I sexually experienced. Bel was right, in this instance—that night I was an eternal virgin.

But I didn't understand any of this back then. After my de-baggaging, I was in so much pain that I believed my body was broken. When Ex-Boyfriend asked me what was wrong—he wasn't so dense that he couldn't sense that something was off—I insisted I was fine. He fell asleep. I didn't sleep at all.

I was probably in shock.

In retrospect.

THE ROMANCE NOVEL is a beautiful genre. That's why, despite these painful virgin tropes, I keep reading them. When they're written well, books about the struggle to find human connection—emotional and physical—are deeply gratifying.

Some readers criticize the predictability of the genre. But, like it does for most genres, predictability makes romance novels more enjoyable, not less. Romance is predictable in the way any genre is predictable: as predictable as a Sherlock Holmes story, as predictable as a sonnet.

"Predictable" simply means that the books share genre conventions to which they must conform and use to tell their stories. These conventions can be constraining, like the quatrains and couplets of a sonnet. But they can also create a freedom within that constraint, as any author of metrical poetry will tell you. Readers appreciate an author who can dazzle from within those conventions.

Any acrobat can flip and twirl. The acrobat who flips and twirls on a tightrope is astounding. The tightrope is the genre with its constraints and conventions.

But here's the other thing about genres: they are allowed to grow and change as the needs of their audiences grow and change.

Wendell and her co-author Candy Tan, in their 2009 book on romance novels, *Beyond Heaving Bosoms*, take on the trope of innocence—usually depicted using virginity—in romance novels of all stripes, not just historicals:

> One of the more peculiar constants of most romance novels, from historicals to contemporaries to paranormals to even erotica, is the sexually unawakened state of the heroine. She's relatively innocent, as proven by her inexperience or her outright virginity. No matter what type she is, she is definitely not the ho-type. Therein lies the deep, humid, dark, and somewhat curious den that is home to the two sacred mythical beasts beloved to Romancelandia. They're interconnected, if you know what we mean (and we think you do): the Unawakened Woman

and the Heroic Wang of Mighty Lovin'. They are the plague and the backbone of romance.

The virginal heroine and heroic wang are long-entrenched conventions of romance novels. But they need to go. They need to go along with the interminable whiteness of the characters of most romance novels, and other sad holdovers.

Romance writers do push genre boundaries. They stay on the tightrope but retrace the conventions in ways that allow for new ways of thinking about sexuality. For readers like me, for rape survivors and abuse survivors, for those of us whose virginity never was ours to begin with—we are grateful.

Courtney Milan's 2011 historical romance novel *Unclaimed* features a virginal leading man, Sir Mark Turner, and a courtesan, Jessica Farleigh, hired to seduce him and destroy his reputation. The book is sexy, conventional (genre-wise), and wound up tight. And yet it flips the virginal heroine trope on its head. That Milan could do all of this and remain on the tightrope only makes her writerly acrobatics more amazing. Milan avoided the plague and maintained the backbone. And with the rest of her novels, she does it over and over. Other writers manage to avoid the plague as well. But they are rare, still.

I KNOW that having sex for the first time is not usually like it is in a romance novel. Even friends who aren't rape survivors have told me that their first time was similar to my de-baggaging. Terrible—painful, with insensitive partners who are snoring before you know it's over.

But usually a girl or woman gets to choose whom she's with when she loses her virginity. I never got to choose. Bel never got to choose. But more than that, we never got to be virgins. From the moment I was aware of my sexuality, I was already not-a-virgin. The first person to press his lips to mine was the first person to stick his dick in me. I didn't know what a condom was, and, no, he didn't use one.

I lost so much that day. Not just my virginity.

It's curious that we say "lose" when we talk about virginity. The language of "lose," of "loss," implies that virginity is something that can be found again. After all, few things are lost forever. The old-fashioned term "ruined" seems far more accurate. Thomas Hardy, ever interested in ruination, wrote a poem called "The Ruined Maid," taking on Victorian notions of virginity and its close bedfellow (heh), ruination.

> *"O 'Melia, my dear, this does everything crown!*
> *Who could have supposed I should meet you in Town?*
> *And whence such fair garments, such pros-per-ity?"—*
> *"O didn't you know I'd been ruined?" said she.*
> *— "You left us in tatters, without shoes or socks,*
> *Tired of digging potatoes, and spudding up docks;*

> *And now you've gay bracelets and bright feathers three!"* —
> *"Yes: that's how we dress when we're ruined,"*
> *said she.*

And on it goes, the poor country girl amazed by the dazzling jewels, dress, and speech of her former counterpart, now "ruined," the reader supposes, by a coincidence of her sexual actions and the rigid moral dictates of society.

What's not mentioned in the poem is that the ruined woman must be well provided for in her new role as a rich man's mistress. Ruination in Victorian society did not immediately mean wealth and education, after all, but it could. And, by the end, it appears that both women—the poor working woman, aged early by her hard life, and the rich man's mistress—are ruined after a fashion. The double meaning of the word "ruined" makes the poem work.

Nevertheless, the line of demarcation is clear. The overworked country girl and the socially ruined mistress are not the same.

A girl does not come back from being ruined. What's lost cannot be found. You just have to pick up the ruined stuff of yourself, and move on. And someday after moving on, someday soon or someday later, you will find that even if you're ruined, *even if you're broken*, you are more than you were before. You are more than what you lost. You are everything you need to be.

7

WHO'S KAY?

I'm thirteen years old and in the mountains of Colorado, and it's cold.

I stuff Tomas's phone number into the pocket of my ski parka. Stepping out of his condominium and into the cold night air, I slide into the warm taxicab. I watch Tomas through the foggy car window as the cab pulls away. He stands barefoot in his doorway in a dark fleece pullover and jeans, his arms wrapped around himself, hopping from foot to foot. I touch the glass, a wave. He doesn't wave back.

He turns back through the doorway, and the door closes.

Riding in silence, I feel like I've lost so much, and yet the worst is still to come. I have lost because Tomas is gone, and I must go back to my family. The cab smells like pizza—there's an open box in the front, the driver's half-eaten dinner. I press my back into the rough vinyl of my seat.

In my feeling of loss, I grasp onto an idea that might save me. I hold onto this hope, suddenly. If I keep hold of this hope, I'll make it through.

The hope—quite simply—is love. I've found love. I'm sure of it. This must be love, what I feel for Tomas. What else could confuse me so much, make me stay out three hours past my curfew? How else to explain the things he said to me? The things he did to me?

How he held my hair back from my face, grasping it at the nape of my neck in one hand, holding my chin with the other, examining my face as though he were a scientist, me a specimen: *You are so beautiful.*

He made me feel like the most beautiful woman in the world.

Woman. Now I'm a woman. I think of the things that have changed in me. I know I'm changed.

The cab drives on the dark mountain highway for what seems like forever but is only twenty minutes according to my watch, and then it exits onto the road that will take me back to where I'm supposed to be. It's late, too late. I'm the only person on the street when the cab drops me in front of the hotel in the middle of the ski village. The normally bustling walkways are deserted.

I take the hotel elevator to our floor and walk down the hall to our room. The hall seems darker than usual, the darkness enhanced by the very late hour, and by the strange dizziness I feel. I slip my key into the lock, missing the first time, dizzy. Finally the door unlocks. I try to open the door quietly. The lights are out, and the room is silent.

My mother doesn't turn to face me when I enter. She feigns sleep in the dark, but I know better. I glance at the time on the red digital clock by the bed. The numbers blaze in my brain—one o'clock. I'm three hours past my curfew.

I'm afraid of what my mother is going to do to me.

I called my mother three times that night, and each time, my mother's voice changed. At ten o'clock, I called her from a payphone near the hot springs to tell her I would be missing my curfew. She sounded furious. I'm never late—I'm too terrified of punishment.

The second time I called her, I used the phone in Tomas's condo. I told her I was fine, and that I would be home soon. On the phone, she sounded afraid, panicked, even when I told her I was safe. It was weird to hear her sound afraid. My mother is never afraid.

I called her a third time just before I left in the cab for the twenty-minute ride back to our hotel. I didn't want her to worry about me. The third time I called, she sounded tired.

After crossing the room, I take off my parka and climb into the rollaway bed. The wheels and springs squeak. I realize I'm shaking. I can't move or think or brush my teeth or wash my face. My world, and my life, seem so far away—the eighth grade and my home back in North Carolina, even my mother in the bed across the room. I'm all alone on that small uncomfortable bed, and I know it.

Things have changed. I'm alone now. Alone. No one will understand what has happened. I have no one to tell: not my mother, not my sister, not my friends at school.

I clutch my secret and try to sleep.

At thirteen, I'm five feet ten inches tall. Men call out to me when I pass them on the street or at the mall. I listen to how they talk and wonder about them—what their complex words imply.

But in middle school, things are different. I rarely receive attention from boys. I'm too tall and can't find clothes like the other girls wear. I'm always reading books and never go to parties. I've never had a boyfriend, never been to a party, never even been kissed.

Until now.

I don't sleep. I don't move, roll over, or even breathe. Breathing, sleeping, eating—all seem foreign, actions done by another girl.

In the morning, my mother is curt like she always is when she's angry with me.

"You're flying home today," she tells me when I get out of the shower.

"What?" I panic. I'm not supposed to leave today. I'm supposed to call Tomas today.

"I've already made the flight arrangements."

I stand in my corner of the room by my rollaway bed. Urgency overwhelms me—I can't leave today, I must see Tomas again. What if I never see him again? I will be alone again, like I am every other day of my life.

"I don't want to go," I say, trying to stay calm, but I know I'm no good at hiding emotion.

"Did you have sex with him?" my mother asks.

"No." I can't tell her the truth. She would never understand. She would only judge me, like she always does.

A few hours later, I ride in the shuttle to the airport. I fly home.

Back home that night, I call my cousin on the phone, a cousin who is more like a big sister to me. I beg her to come to my parents' house, *right now*, I say. We go into the guest room. For some reason, talking about my secret in my own bedroom, with its childish twin beds and awkward memories, feels wrong.

I want to tell my cousin what happened. She's in her early twenties and smart. I need someone to share my secret with. It's burning up inside of me.

"I had sex with Tomas in Colorado," I say.

She asks who he is, how old he is.

I tell her how we met. I say, "He's twenty-four."

She freaks out. "Katie," she says, stumbling over her words. "This is wrong. It's not what you think. This isn't how it's supposed to be." She picks up my hand. "This is rape."

I jerk back from her. It's the first time I hear the word *rape* in a conversation instead of a book. I'm not sure what it means. I just know it means something bad.

"No, he likes me."

"I want to kill him," she says. "He hurt you."

I'm so confused. What he did had hurt, at least I think it had, but I can't remember very much. In fact, it's hard to remember anything.

"Did he use a condom?" my cousin asks.

I look to the side. "What does that mean?"

"You have to tell your parents," she says.

"No, no way," I say. "They'll kill me. My mom will kill me."

She convinces me to do it anyway.

When my mom returns home from Colorado the next day, we gather in our living room, the one with all of the windows that open into the backyard like a fishbowl or a police interrogation room on television. It feels like the entire world can see our conversation, can hear it.

My cousin is there, sitting next to me. I say the words I rehearsed with her. "I had sex with Tomas in Colorado."

Then, the world explodes. They are angry, yelling. So many words at once. I'm embarrassed. I want all of the yelling to stop so I can go back upstairs to my room.

My parents ask the condom question again, this time with more detail. I realize what they mean.

"No," I say.

He didn't use a condom. Those words make them even more angry. My father is pacing around. Then, he goes to the kitchen and makes a phone call.

I feel the dizziness again like I felt that night when I returned to the hotel room. Like there is a world where people live, where my own body moves, but the me of it isn't there anymore.

BEFORE THE TRIP TO COLORADO, ski resorts felt like Disneyland: big, fun, and safe. Vail is the same way, but on a much larger scale. The man I'm chatting with on the chair lift is so hot I want to faint, but he's clearly older than me, so I figure he won't be interested.

"How old are you?" he asks.

I want him to keep talking to me, so I lie about my age: I say I'm fourteen, that I'm in high school. We talk and flirt some more, and then he asks if I want to ski with him for a little while, since we're both skiing alone. I agree. We're a good match in skill. We ski until the chair lifts close, racing to the bottom at five o'clock to catch the last chair up.

Before I can take off down the slope, he says, "Follow me."

He leads me through the trees to the top of a slender trail with small, soft moguls. We stop at the top.

"Look," he says. "Isn't it amazing here?"

I look ahead at the view, at the craggy stone mountains, so different than the green hills of the mountains back home in North Carolina.

"Yes," I say.

He leans over and kisses me. I concentrate on relaxing, since I've never kissed a boy before. I wonder if all boys' faces feel so rough.

"This is your first kiss, isn't it," he says. His words aren't a question. He sounds pleased that I've never kissed anyone before.

I'm too embarrassed to answer.

"Can I see you tonight?" he asks.

"Okay."

When I get back to the hotel after skiing, I tell my mom that I have a date.

"How old is he?" my mom asks.

"Sixteen." I say, even though he told me he's twenty-four. He told me no one would understand. He made me feel so special and safe. He told me everything would be fine.

That night, I follow the directions he gave me, taking a cab to meet him at his condominium.

Before we get into his car, I feel like I should tell him the truth about my own age. I'm nervous, though, because I'm afraid he won't want to go out with me.

"I'm not fourteen," I say, squeezing my hands together.

"How old are you?" he asks.

"I'm thirteen."

"What grade are you in?"

"Eighth." I want to sink into the snowbank in the parking lot. I sound like a little kid.

He smiles. "That's okay," he says. "Come on."

I'm so relieved I want to cry. He still wants to be with me. I'm still special.

We drive up into the hills—not to a restaurant like I was expecting. I've never been on a date before, but I'm pretty sure that dates involve restaurants, dinner, walks, and holding hands.

Tomas parks in a clearing between tall conifer trees. He opens the trunk of the car and takes out a bundle of towels.

"We're at a hot spring," he says, pointing toward a rocky cliff and a pathway leading downhill.

I see other cars parked in the nearby shadows. I can hear a river rushing below the rocky cliff, but it's too dark to see it. Tomas doesn't walk toward that pathway, though. No, he leads me the other way, toward the shadows between the trees and the car.

He spreads a towel on the ground. Then, he pulls me to him and kisses me. I'm still learning how to kiss. I try to follow his lead so I don't make any mistakes.

He lays me down on the towel. He lies on top of me, between my legs. He pulls my sweater off. He pulls my boots and socks and pants off.

It's cold.

I think, It's March in Colorado, on a bare mountaintop in the middle of the night. Of course it is freezing cold.

He kisses my neck.

I stare at the sky, at the bright white moon glowing above the tops of the trees, at the bits of cloud floating there, at the unfathomable number of stars. I think, You can never see so many stars back home on the east coast. Their brightness is always dulled by humidity and urban glare.

I don't know when he pulls off my underwear, but when he pushes himself inside me I scream. I freeze with pain, shock, and fear. I can't move. So he lifts my legs like a Raggedy-Ann doll, no bones, no muscle. I cry.

I cry a lot, I think.

When he's done I take the clothes he hands me and put them on, the clothes of another person, it seems, the clothes of a little girl. I'm embarrassed my panties are so girlish, with frills and low-cut legs, not something a woman would wear.

I stumble and nearly fall, catching myself by leaning against the cold car bumper to pull on my panties.

Panties, such a childish word. A childish word for a child.

AFTER I TELL my parents what happened with Tomas, my father says, "I'm going to catch him and throw him in jail. Tell me everything you know about him."

But I'm hysterical, screaming. My father is angry with me.

"You hurt your mother so much," he says.

"Tomas didn't hurt me," I tell him. "He loves me!"

"He doesn't love you!" my mother yells. "Can't you see?"

I can't see.

I could not see. They could not see. No one could see that where memories should have been, there was nothing.

My mother gets serious. "You can't tell anyone about Tomas," she says. "People will judge you. They'll think badly of you if they know what happened."

I don't understand what she means.

I didn't know the word *slut*, not yet. I would later.

I only had questions: Why shouldn't I be proud that a beautiful man loved me enough to spend an entire night with me, to tell me I'm beautiful, to kiss me? He didn't even mind when I told him I was only thirteen. He loves me how I am, like no one loved me before.

That cold night, after we returned from the hot springs to his condo, he pulled my hair from my face and held it at the nape of my neck. "You are so beautiful," he said. And then he said, "Let's have sex again."

THAT AWFUL DAY, after I told my parents what happened with Tomas and my father made that phone call, here's what I think happened. My memory is fuzzy, but I'll do my best recounting.

To get the facts of what happened, I could ask my parents what they remember. But we don't talk about Tomas in my family. Every time I try to talk about Tomas, things go badly. We all fall into a spiral of guilt.

I feel guilty for hurting them. Sometimes they let me feel guilty. And sometimes that makes me mad.

I'm sure they feel guilty for not protecting me. They've

never said so outright, but I'm a parent now, and I know about that guilt.

Sometimes they want to talk to me about my feelings. I don't want to talk to them about my feelings because, even now, thirty years later, that's still too weird. It's easier to talk to a million strangers in a chapter in a book about my feelings than to look at my parents' faces and do it.

So, I will do the best I can to remember without their help.

As best as I can remember, after my father made that phone call, things went like this.

I remember the emergency clinic. A room. Lots of people coming in and out.

I'm lying on a bed. They treat me as though my case were emergent. As though Tomas didn't rape me days before, but instead minutes before. I remember a vaginal exam, which was the first one of my life. What were they looking for? I don't know. Did they do a rape kit? Were they called rape kits then? I don't know.

I remember needles, shots. I don't know how many. More than one. Less than ten. I think it was less than ten.

They didn't tell me what was happening or why. I don't think they did. Everything was happening so quickly. I think it was quickly. I remember my father, a doctor, being there. I don't remember who else was there. I literally do not remember who else was in the room. Who looked up my vagina. Who stuck me with needles. Who took swabs and samples and drew my blood.

I remember the ceiling tiles and the lights, though. Fluorescent, of course. This was 1990. There was no corporate or industrial lighting that was soothing, not then.

The lighting was all jarring and ugly and full of flickering tubes.

Speculation: The exam table was vinyl and covered in paper. I know about the exam table not because I remember how the table felt but because I've been back to that particular clinic and know what the tables are like.

More speculation: The shots contained antibiotics to kill any diseases he might have given me that could be killed with antibiotics because he didn't use a condom.

The diseases he might have given me that couldn't be killed with antibiotics? That helped explain the terrorized expression on my mother's face. On my father's face.

I didn't get it then.

I'm a mom now. I get it now.

There was blood in their tears. Someone else's blood. Mine.

I REMEMBER BEING RAPED by Tomas now. I'm still angry about what he did to me. I'm angry that I never got to be a virgin, not really. I'm angry that I've always had a screwed-up relationship with sex and probably always will.

He raped me on April 1st of my eighth grade year. The following autumn, I started high school. High school was hard for me—not the classes, not the sports. Not the usual stuff—everything else.

I showed up at a new school full of new people who hadn't known me before. They hadn't known the awkward, ugly, nerdy me from middle school. They didn't have those associations. No thick glasses, no braces. No awkward growth spurt that took me from five-two to five-ten in a matter of months. When I arrived at high school, I had so much to learn about being a person boys wanted to talk to.

The first weekend of high school, I learned that I had nice legs. I learned that piece of information from a senior boy, Luke, who was happy to take my pants off, and I, not knowing any better, was happy to let him. I thought that taking our clothes off together meant he would be my boyfriend.

On Monday, when the senior boy, Luke, wouldn't say hi to me in the hallway, I was hurt and confused. So I asked my new friend, a sophomore named Alice, why Luke had ignored me. Alice and I sat on a bench together, heads huddled so no one else could hear.

"Why won't Luke talk to me?" I asked.

"You guys hooked up," Alice said.

What I wanted to say: What does "hooked up" mean? And why does that mean he won't talk to me?

Instead of saying the words, I drew an inference about what the phrase meant. I didn't want my new friend at my new school to think I was an idiot.

I tried to think of a question to ask Alice that would help me understand Luke's meanness without sounding too naive.

"So guys don't talk to girls they hook up with?"

"Well, it's not like there are rules," Alice said, sounding wise. "But you don't have to talk to people you hook up with. It's not like you're dating or anything."

What I wanted to know: How do you find out when you are dating?

"Honestly," Alice said, "Haven't you done this before?"

Correct answer: I didn't know.

I might not have been a virgin sitting on that bench with Alice, but I was still a naive child.

―――――

I DIDN'T EVEN REMEMBER what Tomas did to me, not exactly, until two years after it happened, during the darkest part of winter my sophomore year of high school.

I was lying on a friend's bed—a sensitive girl, one of my closest friends in high school. Miriam.

Miriam told me about being attacked by a man in a neighbor's swimming pool, and how she just barely escaped him. I pictured her legs kicking desperately in the nighttime lights of a swimming pool, the shadows that her desperation would have cast in the water. How her fingers would have grabbed at the concrete edge and pulled herself free of the water. How she would have run.

Hearing Miriam's words, how this man had attacked her, triggered something in me. Suddenly, my memories escaped whatever trap had been meant to protect a thirteen-year-old girl. Those memories sprang free.

At first, the memories were only bits and pieces. I remembered fear and nausea. I remembered cold and nakedness. I remembered fire, awful, painful fire. I remembered I was supposed to be someplace else but I couldn't get there.

I remember he kept handing me quarters for the payphone. Telling me to call my mom. Telling me to say I'm okay.

On Miriam's bed, I felt cold, as if naked on the ground,

on a small towel with pine needles poking through and sticking my back and shoulders. I could see the sky again, all those stars.

The sky spins. I'm dizzy. I can smell him and feel him burning me. He says a name, but it's not my name—he calls me Kay.

Who's Kay? I think.

Kay must be me.

Tomas didn't just fuck me on that towel. He fucked me up entirely.

KIDS IN MY HIGH SCHOOL, like many high school kids back then, liked to listen to certain songs deemed "classic rock." One of those songs was "Brown Eyed Girl" by Van Morrison. They played that song incessantly. The girl Alice, the one who explained the rules about hooking up to me, danced to it whenever it came on, with her awkward knock-knees and her fingers snapping. I used to dance with her.

Today, I *hate* that song. If it comes on in a café or bar, I'll walk out the door and wait on the sidewalk until it's over.

When I was thirteen and fourteen years old—before that night with Miriam—I loved the song. I'd listen to Morrison singing how hard it was to find his way, but then he saw her—just the other day—and he thought, *My, how you have grown.*

He sang, *Cast my memory back there, Lord / Sometime I'm overcome thinking about / Making love in the green grass / Behind the stadium / With you.*

And I used to want Tomas to come find me, to rescue me from my mundane life, to say to me, *My, how you have grown*.

I would think about having sex outside under the explosion of stars with Tomas, by the hot spring—how romantic, I would think. How lucky I was to have had my first time be there, in that place.

I told the story of my night with Tomas to my high school friends, late at night, in secret. And I didn't think about words like *slut*, or *rape*, or *hookup*. I didn't think anything about my story was strange or weird. And no one told me it was, although thinking about it now, I'm pretty sure they told each other.

The high school boys who fancied themselves in love with me would play "Brown-Eyed Girl" for me on their stereos, thinking they could woo me and my brown eyes.

But while the boys my own age would try to woo me, I would dream of the man who stripped me naked in a Colorado forest and fucked me without a condom.

And then came that night with Miriam.

And the next time someone played "Brown-Eyed Girl," I thought, *Why would Tomas need to say "My how you have grown" to me if he hadn't been fucking a child?*

There are some things that aren't described in Van Morrison's song.

The trying to get dressed afterward.

The sitting on the cold car bumper and pulling on your little-girl underwear that no one has ever seen before except your mommy.

The embarrassment you feel because you're certain that

you've done it, it meaning sex, wrongly because you cried and everything hurt.

The shaking of your body, every bone, every finger and toe, and not from the cold. No, you're shaking like you have a fever, like you might die but you aren't sure why.

Why can't I stop shaking? I can't get my foot into my underwear, and he's watching me. I'm so embarrassed and I'm going to cry again. Why? Why am I crying?

I hate "Brown-Eyed Girl." I have no happy memories of young love and waterfalls to reminisce about. Tomas tainted them all.

EVEN NOW, decades later, part of me still hates myself for fantasizing about Tomas when I was young. I have trouble forgiving myself for defending him to my cousin. For believing that I loved him. For not running away screaming. For not fighting him. For not telling my mom where I was when I called her, or begging her for help—after all, wasn't I in danger? And after, how could I yearn for him, or fantasize about him, if he hurt me so badly?

Even thinking about these feelings, the memories of these feelings, makes me sad for the girl I was. These memories still have the power to make me feel ashamed, even now, after all of the work I've done as an attorney, writer, and activist. Still, even now, the feelings I felt for Tomas when I was thirteen and fourteen years old make me flinch. Make me blame myself. Make a small part of me angry at myself.

And then, after the shame, the blame, and the anger

dissipate, all I can do is acknowledge that what I felt was real, and there's nothing I can do but accept it.

HERE IS the only thing that gives me peace: A man like Tomas would select a victim in a calculating fashion. He was so calculating, in fact, that I likely never had a chance.

Under the bright blue Colorado sky, a man like Tomas would stand in the lift line, and he would look for a girl who was young and alone. And he would figure out a way to ride the chair lift with her. Letting others go ahead of him, if necessary, so that he could sit with her.

It might take a few trips up the chair lift before he found her. The right girl.

He would select a girl who's on vacation so that she's isolated from her support systems, if she has support systems at all. On vacation, she would be far from the places she knows well. She would be disoriented.

He would ask the girl questions to determine whether she would be a good victim. A good victim would have low self-esteem—so he would give her compliments, and see how she reacts. Does she accept the compliments as her due? Or do they make her blush and fret, as though she's never received them before?

A good victim would be socially awkward. She would have few friends; she wouldn't be popular. He would ask about her friends, and see how she describes them. He would say, "You must be really popular back home," and he would see how she responds.

A good victim would be abused or neglected by her

family, either emotionally or physically. So he would ask about her family, and watch her face carefully. Does she trust her parents? Does she share her secrets with them? Do they hurt her?

A good victim would have a mental illness or another disability. She would have a poor ability to make good decisions, to set boundaries, and to assess risks. So he would test for all of these things.

How old are you?

Follow me.

This is your first kiss, isn't it.

The only thing that gives me peace is this: Before we ever left the snow, he'd already selected his victim.

THESE DAYS, among other things, I work as an activist in the arena of sexual assault and violence. I often give interviews to journalists who are writing stories about activists, survivors, rape policy, or any other topic that they think I might have insight about.

Recently, I gave an interview to a college student. Her media request came to a person who handles such things for me, and it came to me with the message that I didn't have to give the interview if I didn't want to—a college student might not be worth my time.

But I didn't mind doing the interview. I figured not many people would take the time to talk to this young person. But as she was an aspiring journalist doing important work, I felt she deserved my time as much as *The New Republic* or *The New York Times*.

During our phone call, the young journalist asked me about being raped and being a rape advocate. These were questions I was accustomed to. Then she asked me this: "What have you done to heal after being raped?"

Unexpectedly, I laughed. I was embarrassed by my inappropriate reaction. "I'm sorry I laughed," I said. "No one has ever asked me that question before."

At that point, the girl and I had been talking for a while, and she'd overcome her initial shyness of me. "Do you talk about being raped with anyone? Like, counseling?"

No, not really, I thought. *I never talk about it with my therapist. Actually, now that I think about it, that's really weird.*

"No. I don't think I've ever done anything to help me heal after being raped," I said, and the words seemed true.

After we hung up, I sat down on my comfortable couch in my comfortable home and wondered why.

Why haven't I done anything to heal? I wondered. *How can I reach back so many years and repair what's broken?*

And that's when I realized I was approaching the question all wrong.

You can't go back. You can't fix what was broken ten years, twenty years, or thirty years ago. All you can do is learn to carry the burden. And as the years go by, the burden gets lighter and lighter, until it's part of you, and it's no longer burden at all.

It becomes a strength—you've made it one.

I've spent thirty years healing, actually. Thirteen-year-old me is still sick with pain and sadness, and she always will be. But I'm here to comfort her, and to keep her safe.

Who's Kay?

Kay is me.

8

NIGHTMARE ROOM

I find out about the art installation, ironically, outside of a favorite coffee shop.

An acquaintance who works at the art museum asks me about the installation. "Have you been to see it?" She sounds excited to hear my answer.

"What installation?" I say. "What are you talking about?"

She's taken aback by my surprise. She thought for sure I knew about it. She thought I would be thrilled to be featured in the groundbreaking installation for which the artist secretly videoed strangers in coffeeshops.

"Didn't you sign a release?" She seems worried, brows drawn together above her honest face.

"No, I didn't sign a release."

Before she mentioned the installation, we were chatting, two acquaintances catching up. Smiling with her that morning, I felt the day opening up before me like the expanse of the table at the coffee shop where my laptop sat, ready for me to write.

Now, I'm not smiling. My arms are crossed over my chest. I feel like I'm closing in on myself. Even my body knows that something has gone gravely wrong. I need to figure out exactly what has gone wrong, and exactly how, so I know what I need to do to make things right again.

"Tell me everything," I say, trying to seem calm.

She describes the installation to me. As she speaks, I can see that she's also trying to keep the conversation normal, as though what's happening between us hasn't moved into the realm of the bizarre. As though she isn't describing a video clip of my face projected on a loop at a museum.

"The installation is called *Dream Rooms*," she says.

"What does it look like?" I ask. "How large is it?" I ask. "Where is it displayed, exactly?" I ask. I want to know all of the details, as though the details might soothe me.

The details don't soothe me. I'm trying to hide my panic, here on the patio of a local coffee shop, where I've abandoned my laptop and purse inside and don't care at all. I don't want this acquaintance to think that I'm overreacting to what she is saying to me.

But I'm deeply worried.

What I learn from her: Video footage of my face, captured by a stranger at a coffee shop at some point in the past, enlarged to the size of a picture window, is projected on the wall just inside the main entrance of the North Carolina Museum of Art. Footage of others is projected alongside me. Maybe I'm one of a dozen? She isn't sure. The projection is on a loop. Over and over, my face. Projected.

"What do I look like?" I ask.

"You look pretty," she says quickly, as though my prettiness would reassure me.

"Am I wearing glasses? What about my hair?"

With these questions, I'm trying to figure out when the video was taken. I don't wear glasses anymore. I've grown out my hair.

She doesn't recall the details. *But she remembers that I'm pretty*, I think, doubting her compliment, now.

"I'm sorry I told you," she blurts, sensing my obvious distress. "Please don't be worried."

I'm not sorry she told me. I would rather know things, even if they hurt.

THERE'S a theory in law called the thin skull doctrine. It goes like this. When you injure someone, you're responsible for the injuries that you cause, even if the person you injure is more vulnerable to harm than an average person might be. For example, if you punch someone in the face who has a brittle bone disorder, you are responsible if their cheekbone shatters, sustaining more damage than a person would who didn't have the disorder. In short, you must "take your victims as you find them."

You can imagine the gruesome history of how the rule got its name—the crash of a carriage, a gravely injured woman, and a lawsuit.[1]

The points is, because we can't always be aware of the harm we might cause to other people, we must be careful with the people we live among. I've always liked the thin skull doctrine, despite its grisly name, because I believe it encourages us to take care. It reminds us that we never know how fragile others might be, or how much others might be suffering, just under the surface of their skin.

AFTER MY ACQUAINTANCE tells me about the installation with the video of my face, all I want to do is see it. No: what I feel is more than mere want. I *need* to see it. I can't work. I can't think about anything else. I can do nothing except try to find out more about it.

Perhaps the installation won't be as bad as I imagine. Perhaps, it will be nothing.

After my acquaintance leaves—her face marked by uncertainty—I dash back into the coffee shop, back to my laptop, and search the installation online. Is my picture on the internet, taken by this artist? Did he publish video of me online?

I find the installation's webpage on the website of the museum. The webpage has a still photo of the installation along with a description and the statement of purpose. The still photo doesn't feature my face, but instead the faces of four other strangers. I wonder if any of the other four know that their faces are projected on the wall at the museum. I wonder if they signed releases.

I read the description.

> *Over the course of its 19 minutes, "Dream Rooms" shows 28 people, four at a time. While none of the subjects are in anything like a compromising position, they all appear to*

be deeply engrossed with whatever is on their computer screens.

I am one of twenty-eight people. I do the math: dividing twenty-eight by four makes seven arrays of videoed strangers, one of them me. Dividing nineteen minutes by seven means that there is a two-minute, forty-two-second video clip of me projected on the wall at the museum.

I wonder at the word "compromising," and the phrase, "compromising position." As a person who works with words, I think about how the word "compromising" has changed over the years, decades, centuries. How what was considered compromising, even in my mother's time, was so different than what is considered compromising today.

I wonder why the museum decided to tell readers that the video doesn't depict people who are compromised, why they bothered to mention it at all. Why would anyone think that we are? Unless, when you are videoed against your will, you always are?

We who are in the installation against our will are not "in anything like a compromising position" in the opinion of the museum, or the artist, but how do they know? I think of how a woman might have left her husband, or a daughter might have hidden from her father, and now he, whichever he, would know where she is and what she is doing if he were to see her in the video. I think of how easy it is to compromise a person's position when you don't know how fragile a person's position is.

I think of the word "position," when paired with the word "compromising," and how together, these days, they are lewd. And I wonder if the museum paired them in this way on purpose, to put the idea of the illicit in viewers' brains deliberately. I think of photographs of politicians caught in compromising positions. Of blackmail. Of careers destroyed by compromising positions.

I think I do not want to have anything to do with the phrase *compromising position*.

NEXT, I read the artist's statement.

> *Dream Rooms examines our wired world of the 21st century. Individuals are seen in coffee shops, wholly absorbed, their trancelike states brought on primarily through an intense engagement with the alternate reality presented by laptops and smart phones.*

My first thought, what I'm able to think with the part of my brain that isn't in a panic, is that the artist's statement is so pretentious that it reads like a satire of an artist's statement. My second thought is that I can never go to a coffee shop again.

The part of my brain that is in a panic reads the word "trancelike" again and again, wondering who selected that word, the artist or the museum or someone else entirely. And I wonder if the writer knows what the word "trance" means—if they've ever looked it up in a dictionary. There's the mystical meaning, yes. But then there's the other meaning, the one that doctors use.

I wonder if the person who wrote this passage has ever been in a trance, has ever been half-conscious and unable to respond to external stimuli. If they've ever seen, or been, someone harmed enough to have been put into a trancelike state. Impossible, I think.

No one who has been harmed that badly, or been close to someone who has, could have written that paragraph. Could have been associated with Dream Rooms.

My eye keeps tracking back to the still photo of the installation. A grid of four faces. Somewhere, one of those faces is mine.

———

THE THIN SKULL doctrine states that when a person is injured, the injured person's invisible vulnerability to harm is not a defense that the injurer can use.

In my life, men have done horrible things to my body, things that have made me feel that my body was not my own. They have made me question where the world ends and my body begins, as though I do not have the same rights to my skin, my hands, my hair, my face, as other humans have to theirs. As *men* have to theirs. No, as *white men* have to theirs.

When I was in the eighth grade, a man raped me in a forest.

When I was a freshman in college, an older student stalked me. He would wait outside my dorm room, sit in our dorm common room, follow me from building to building. He let me know he had access to firearms. Eventually, after another student witnessed the stalking, he —an athlete on scholarship—risked everything to make the stalker stop. I never asked how he did it.

Later, when I was still in school, a married professor tried to start a sexual relationship with me, and I rejected him. I feared, reasonably, that the aftermath would cost me my degree, and maybe my career. The professor's wife threatened to sue me for ruining her marriage. I had to hire an attorney to protect me.

When I was still in school, a friend raped me after we went out to a bar together. He pinned me down with his elbow across the back of my skull. Earlier, we spent the evening drinking martinis, flirting, having a lovely time. All I could think, for days and weeks after, was, *How can we tell when we are in danger? How can we ever tell when we are safe?*

My stories are awful, but they are not unique. I was talking to my friend recently about being raped in graduate school, about the martinis and the bar on Franklin Street. She said, *Me too.* And then she said, *Which bar on Franklin Street is* your *bar?*

When I read the description of Dream Rooms I wondered, *Which coffee shop?*

———

MOMENTS AFTER LEARNING that my face is part of an installation, I need to understand everything about it. I'm obsessed. I can't transport myself from Chapel Hill to the interior of the North Carolina Museum of Art in Raleigh, in part because it is closed that day, Monday. Instead, I call my husband and tell him everything. He says he'll take me tomorrow, Tuesday. I realize, after speaking with him, that going with someone else is a good idea. Driving there alone

—as much as I want, no, need, to see the installation—is not a good idea.

I know what I'm feeling. My heart is beating quickly. My hands are shaking. I'm blinking too much. I know what all of these things mean. Any diagnostician with the most basic skills would know what these things mean. They would mean I shouldn't drive a car. They would mean I'm having a traumatic reaction. I'm lucky, I tell myself, that the day is Monday and the museum is closed.

I read more of the description of the installation on the museum's website.

> *... Dream Rooms seek[s] to lay bare the effects of technologically mediated intimacy and chronic multitasking. ... How does the idea of surveillance alter our experience of these individuals? Each character is intimately examined in public space, comfortably anonymous and secure in the privacy of his or her thoughts and behavior, while the gaze of the camera records impulses and reactions.*

My eyes stick on certain words in the description:

Bare.
Intimacy.
Relationship.
Surveillance.
Experience.
Character
Intimate.
Examine.

Privacy.
Gaze.
Impulses.

I am bare. I have been surveilled, intimately. My privacy is no more. I have been experienced, gazed upon. One man's impulse to intimately examine me has taken precedence over my bodily autonomy, my privacy. I'm no longer a person, merely a character, recorded.

Where does my body end and his gaze begin?

I'm sick. I need to vomit. I run to the bathroom of the coffee shop. I stand in a stall, door locked. I'm not sure what to do. Do I call my husband for help?

No, that's ridiculous. He's at work. You don't need help.

Emerging from the bathroom, I realize that, in my panic, I've left my purse and laptop alone again, and I feel lucky they haven't been stolen.

Arms crossed over my middle, I make my way back to my seat. I look around me at the coffee shop where I am working, suddenly afraid. I know that my fear is irrational. But I feel it anyway. I look around me, *Is someone watching me now? Am I safe?* I don't know how to reconcile all of the words of Dream Rooms with where I'm sitting now.

I pack my bag. My hands, they're shaking.

I drive home.

Inside, I shut the blinds.

All I want to do is go to the museum and see the installation for myself. I think, *If I can only see it for myself then I will see it isn't as bad as I am imagining.*

Surely this installation isn't as bad as I am imagining it

to be. It can't be as bad as it seems from what I'm reading. It isn't possible.

No one would use us, use me, like that. Who would use us, use me, like that?

I research the artist.

His name: William Noland. He is a white man in late middle age, or so I could see from his portrait. He's a professor of art at Duke University, a wealthy private university here in the part of North Carolina where I live.

I know a lot about Duke University because I went there for my undergraduate degree. And I know a lot about how higher education works because I'm a professor and have been one, more or less, since I was in my late twenties.

Because I know about Duke University and about higher education, I know that Noland makes his living by getting his art shown in art museums. Museums don't necessarily pay him directly—Duke does that. The North Carolina Museum of Art, by selecting Dream Rooms to exhibit, has justified Noland's employment by Duke.

In a similar fashion, law reviews didn't pay me to publish my articles, but those articles helped justify my employment as a law professor. That's how academia works. We, the professors, prove our worth to our institutions through external validation of our expertise. If you're an artist and you need external validation of your value, you need museums to show your art.

My face, monstrously projected on the walls of the North Carolina Museum of Art, has indirectly paid Noland's salary.

I think what kind of security in yourself, in your wealth, in your whiteness and maleness, in your power and privilege, it would take to secretly video people, even if they weren't in *compromising positions*, and sell that video as art. I can't imagine what it would take to sit in a coffee shop and seek out, on purpose, the most vulnerable people around me, and turn on my camera.

And to do so in order to use *the idea of surveillance* to *alter our experience of these individuals?* I can't even imagine what kind of freedom from retribution it would take to do such a thing.

Imagine being so unafraid. Imagine being so unworried. Imagine. Imagine having so little fear of the wrath of others that you would video them, on purpose, to expose their vulnerabilities.

Before it happened to me, I couldn't imagine such a thing.

Noland, in his artist statement, says that he preyed on my immersion in my writing, on my obliviousness to my surroundings. But he's wrong. I wasn't oblivious at all.

No. I made a deliberate decision to do what I did, to be where I was.

What Noland preyed on was my trust in the people I was working near.

It took so long for me to build that trust. I work so hard to maintain it. And Noland, with his cavalier attitude and little video camera, broke my trust in, quite literally, everyone around me.

WHEN YOU'VE SURVIVED TRAUMA, you might develop posttraumatic stress disorder. I did.

PTSD makes it hard for me, and anyone like me, to believe that I will be safe in situations that others take for granted will be safe.

Here's what it takes for me to immerse myself in my work in a coffee shop.

First, I have to leave the house. Some days, leaving the house is hard. Those days, fortunately, have become rare.

Next, I have to find a public place that feels familiar enough that I trust I will be safe there. For years, even in these safe places, I couldn't sit with my back to the room, only to the wall. In the past few years, I've grown able to sit with my back to the room.

Finally, I can only allow myself to grow immersed in my work once I've grown to trust the people around me. I can't, for example, immerse myself in my work on an airplane seated next to a stranger. I can when I'm seated next to my husband. I can't when I'm in a strange city seated alone in a restaurant or coffee shop, but I can if a good friend is there. The people matter, too. I can be in a familiar place, but if there is a stranger who makes me uncomfortable, I will leave.

I can no longer immerse myself in my work in the coffee shop where Dream Rooms was filmed.

———

On the Tuesday after I find out about Dream Rooms, my husband, M., drives me to see it at the North Carolina Museum of Art in Raleigh.

We enter the museum through the main entrance. The main entrance to the museum is bunker-like, all cement protrusions and dark glass, built at the height of brutalism. I realize I'm shaking as we descend the stairs, and I have trouble gripping the handrail. I thread my hand through my husband's elbow, squeezing his arm for stability. Directly ahead of the main staircase, there is a temporary wall, as tall as the gallery, fifteen feet, maybe more. Centered in front of the wall there is a small black bench. And projected onto the wall is Dream Rooms.

We sit on the bench. We wait.

M. holds my hand.

The projection changes every few minutes—*two minutes, forty-two seconds*—but the time feels like eternity. The videos appear in sets of four, two vertical by two horizontal, four strangers, all videoed at coffee shops I recognize, places I frequent. I'm a writer. I work in coffee shops.

I see Caffe Driade of Chapel Hill, mostly. I wonder, for a moment, whether the owners of the coffee shops would mind if they knew that Noland had made these videos of their patrons.

If I were the owner, I would have minded.

And then, suddenly, there I am. My face is in the bottom-right quadrant. I can tell from the video that it was shot a few years ago. Before I had my eye surgery, so I'm still wearing glasses. I still have bangs and short hair. I'm at Caffe Driade. I remember the table. He must have been sitting not five feet from me.

I'm wearing a necklace that used to belong to my grandmother, my father's mother, before she died—my mom had it made for her, a gold disc with my name and birthday etched on the surface. The disc reflects light like a star on my chest. I'm looking down for the entire duration of the video, typing on my computer. I wonder what I'm working on, what *she* is working on, the me who is not me.

Suddenly, I get a chill.

I start to cry.

"How could he," I say.

M. squeezes my hand. He's a calm dude. It's why I picked him, of all of the people on the planet, to spend my life with. But he is not okay with Dream Rooms. "I don't like this," he says. "This is not okay."

Coming from M., these are fierce words.

"Take my picture," I say, handing him my phone.

I stand in front of the projection of myself and have M. take my picture. I want to preserve the scale. I want people to understand how massive this projection is. I'm six feet tall, yet I'm dwarfed by this video projection. I look at the photo after M. takes it. Projection-Katie is bright and clear. Real-life Katie is cast in shadow.

I'm a shaking mass of fear, anxiety, and anger. I try to peel the feelings apart, but I can't. I'm furious that William Noland makes a living from the faces of strangers. I'm furious that the museum put this installation up in the first place. I'm terrified that I will never feel comfortable in public again. I feel naked, exposed.

I don't understand how anyone could have felt differently.

Maybe I have a thin skull. But that's not my fault. And I know I'm not the only one. Of twenty-eight people, statistically speaking, I can't be the only one.

―――

THINGS HAPPEN QUICKLY.

I email the curator of the museum and ask for the installation to be taken down. The curator never replies, not even to give me some pat nonsense about artistic license.

So I do what we do in the early twenty-first century to get responses from organizations that ignore us. I write about how I feel about Dream Rooms on my blog.

> *To the creep who videoed me and called it art:*
> *I don't want to be surveilled, but I didn't have a choice.*
> *I don't want to be experienced, but I didn't have a choice of that either.*
> *I don't want to be intimately examined, but I don't have a choice of that.*
> *I'm not secure, or private.*
> *The gaze of the camera has shattered my feelings of security and privacy.*
> *That's the male artist's privilege. And my female body is now a stranger's to consume.*
> *Again.*

And then I share the blog essay on social media.

Social media gets the reaction that my email to the curator does not. In fact, social media reacts so strongly to the idea that a man could spy on people in vulnerable positions—by his own admission, in the description of the work—and call it art.

Suddenly, on social media, the North Carolina Museum of Art is apologetic about the installation. Suddenly, representatives from the museum want to talk with me. They ask me to contact them privately.

I don't want to talk. There is nothing to discuss. But I agree.

The curator apologizes to me. They're deeply sorry. They're going to take the installation down. I feel a little bit better, not much, but a little bit. The fear I feel, the anxiety, the heightened sense of danger don't go away when the installation goes away. I can't stop thinking about Dream Rooms, the artist who believed what he did was not only right, but good, and the museum curators who agreed with him.

Then things get weird.

All I wanted was for the installation to go away. But I should have known. Compromising positions—even when you swear that they aren't compromising—always attract attention.

A television news reporter from our local CBS affiliate sends me a message.

> **CBS Guy**: I saw your post and wanted to see if you were available and interested to talk on camera today about what happened?
> **Me**: I appreciate your interest in the story. I'm not interested in being on camera. Best of luck.

A conversation ensues in which I advise him about ways he can run the story without me. But he's persistent.

> **CBS Guy**: There's no way I can convince you, right?

Me: No thanks. Part of the problem has to do with how much I do not like being on video.

That's what I wrote, even though it wasn't exactly true. How do I explain to him that the problem isn't about being on video—I do video interviews, video presentations, podcasts, and more.

The problem is that I want to tell my story. My face is me. My words are me. And I know, from the last time I was interviewed on television, how badly things can go.

I already feel raw and exposed. The last thing I want to do is put myself at the mercy of a news crew.

I feel so out of control.

Everything has been stripped away.

I shut the blinds.

AFTER THE INSTALLATION is taken down, I wonder why I don't feel better, why things aren't *back to normal*. I wonder why I'm so angry, still. Questions run through my head. Most of them start with "why."

I write another blog essay, this time with questions.

> *Why did this exhibit go up in the first place?*
> *How did an exhibit full of video of people taken without their permission slip through the museum's curatorial board?*
> *If they don't want the exhibit now, why did they want it then?*
> *Did they just presume the artist had releases?*

> *Are we so inured to the idea that we can video other people that we are not unsettled by this exhibit at all?*

I know it's too late to stop me from being hurt, but maybe it isn't too late to stop someone else from being hurt in the future. I'm trying to cross the line between victim and activist. I don't want to be a victim, only.

WEEKS LATER, a reporter from the Raleigh newspaper contacts me for an interview. I start to wonder if I've fallen into a new, larger loop, one that I'll never emerge from, where Dream Rooms is inside the loop with me and I can't get away from it. A Nightmare Room.

I decline the interview, telling the journalist that everything he needs from me I've already said on my blog. I forget about the phone call.

I forget until the article comes out, at which point I wonder which of my two professions—lawyer or journalist—should be hated more. As I read the article, I feel hate for the journalist, and I feel hate for everyone he interviewed, people from the museum, and lawyers, and Noland himself. I know my hatred is unreasonable, but I feel it anyway.

The article is a puff piece about Noland and the museum. It portrays me as a thin-skinned writer whose feelings got hurt, who overreacted and sicced the Twitter hordes on the museum.

Earlier this fall, an exhibit at the N.C. Museum of Art abruptly disappeared several months ahead of schedule.

The journalist, with his first sentence and his choice of verb and adverb, removes all actors, all causation. Dream Rooms "disappeared"!

No. Dream Rooms is not a magician's coin. It did not disappear. The museum took it down. They made a decision; there was a reason for their decision.

A self-described java junkie, Noland spends lots of time in coffee shops doing what many people do in such settings: staring at a computer screen, oblivious to the surroundings.

See? Noland is a normal guy. He's a "java junkie," according to the journalist. The alliteration makes Noland seem so adorable and harmless. The journalist lets so much about Noland slide.

So Noland began surreptitiously filming people entranced by their computer screens.

Yes, this is completely normal. The java junkie who works at his computer a lot began filming people in secret, and this behavior is, apparently, completely fine.

As I read the article, I wonder how everyone seems to think that Noland's behavior is completely fine. I wonder if I am, indeed, the crazy one.

The end result was "Dream Rooms," which was destined

to be part of a wave of controversial found-art artifacts—a growing trend.

Here, my eye catches on the word "controversial." So much is enclosed in that word.

Controversial is a word that has a meaning. It denotes sides turned (contra) against (verso) one another. But in Dream Rooms, what are the sides? One side's desire to secretly video a person to further his career? And another side's desire to feel safe in public?

Why not name the sides?

The journalist does name them, but he names them wrongly, especially mine.

One of its unwitting subjects discovered she was in it. That was Katie Rose Guest Pryal, a writer from Chapel Hill, and she began registering strong objections starting with an email of protest to the museum.

I "registered strong objections," apparently. I sent an "email of protest." (I didn't.)

And (worst of all) I engaged in Twitter call-out culture, the horrible mob rule that destroys reputations:

Pryal (who declined to be interviewed) also took her complaint to Twitter, where the consensus among her followers was that "Dream Rooms" was "Scary & creepy." In response, the museum issued an apology and canceled "Dream Rooms."

The responses on social media were so much more

nuanced than "scary & creepy." They were overwhelming, and they were supportive. Twitter is a community, a living place, the *only* place where I could find anyone to help me understand what was happening to me.

In the discussions on Twitter, not everyone agreed with one another. Some pointed out that what Noland did was legal—in fact, I was one of those people. I'm a lawyer, after all, which the journalist fails to mention in his article.

No, in this space, this Nightmare Room, I'm merely a "writer from Chapel Hill," Noland's "unwitting subject."

Unwitting, another word that has a meaning: *not aware of the full facts.*

Compared to Noland, the museum curator, and the lawyer the journalist interviewed, I am no one.

As a lawyer, I know Noland broke no laws. That doesn't mean that what he did was ethical. It only means that Noland has a broken sense of right and wrong. And he's not the only one.

> *"I really didn't think it would be an issue and did not think twice about it," said Linda Dougherty, the museum's curator of contemporary art. "We were surprised but also wanted to be considerate of (Pryal's) feelings."*

The museum people were "surprised." They wanted to be "considerate." They were concerned about my "feelings." Ethics—right and wrong—didn't enter into their decision-making at all.

"She found it extremely upsetting and we did not want to keep it up if it was going to cause that much distress."

When I first read the curator's sentence, I doubt myself. All of the voices of support I received—for a moment, none of them matter.

Here, printed on the pages of the major newspaper of my state's capital, spoken by the curator of my state's museum, are words that imply that a thin-skinned but social-media-savvy whiner in Chapel Hill caused them to take the installation down.

Words matter.

The curator could have said her words so many other ways.

"She found it extremely upsetting."

Another way: "We realized that Noland's secret video project was inherently upsetting."

"We did not want to keep it up if it was going to cause that much distress."

Another way: "Because the installation is inherently distressing, we took it down."

Words matter, so much.

The curator said the word "if." She said that I "found it" upsetting. Her words mean that problem was me, not Dream Rooms.

The journalist doesn't question the museum's version of

the story. The journalist makes the museum's version the story of record.

The journalist had access to my version of the story via my blog essays. And I know the journalist read my blog essays, not only because he quotes them, but because the story he wrote rebuts specific arguments I made in those essays.

> *In the case of "Dream Rooms," no money changed hands*
> *—the museum did not pay Noland for the film.*

Perhaps, in my blog essays, I was too oblique about how Noland made money off of Dream Rooms. Perhaps the museum thought it was really important that they defend themselves about the money thing. Perhaps Noland wanted the same.

Whatever the case, the journalist felt it necessary to prove the point about money. But that is not the only defense the journalist mounts.

> *Noland said he would sit at a coffee-shop table with his*
> *camera out in plain sight. When someone sat across from*
> *him, he'd turn it on.*

Why specify that the camera was in plain sight? Does the visibility of the camera alleviate some of Noland's guilt? What difference does it make that the camera was in plain sight if what Noland did was perfectly legal—he could have been wearing a hidden camera, right?

By telling us the camera was in plain sight, Noland—

and the journalist—are shifting blame onto the subjects of the video.

We should have been paying attention.

We should have noticed the camera.

It was our fault.

As I finish the article, I realize what a defense of Noland and the art museum the article really is, and how the journalist portrayed me as a hysterical female who needed to be appeased.

I'm suffering again, this time for standing up for myself all those months before.

Why bother, I wonder. *Why, when it always makes things worse?*

The journalist describes in detail Noland's goals and artistic process, how what he did was not only legal, but also part of a long line of artists pushing artsy boundaries.

> *"Dream Rooms" is one of several recent cases where issues of surveillance, privacy and copyright bump up against each other.*

The lawyer that the journalist interviewed helpfully points out that what Noland did was totally legal.

> *"There is some discomfort from feeling spied upon … But that doesn't make it unlawful."*

The more I read, the more I realize the subtext of the entire article: What the museum did when it took down Dream Rooms was a huge favor for me, and I'm supposed to feel grateful.

It becomes clear that the museum does not believe there was any inherent wrongness in what Noland did.

After the museum canceled "Dream Rooms," it was replaced with "Occulted"—a similarly styled Noland film about London as the most heavily surveilled place on earth.

Dream Rooms was filled with people who were local. The replacement installation was filled with people from London. It was doubtful that someone would wander in and complain if they had to hop on a plane to do so.

"I tried to pick people who looked like I could identify with."

When I read these words of Noland's, I feel scared again. Noland picked me on purpose. I wasn't random. I was *targeted*. He thought he identified with me.

I want to take a shower. To scrub my skin, to scrub his eyes off of my body.

Noland was distressed to learn of Pryal's reaction to "Dream Rooms," so he did not object to the film being taken down. But he believes the larger point of the work remains valid.

I have changed nothing. Nothing has changed. Nothing will change.

"We're being watched."

Maybe. But Noland is the one who videoed twenty-eight people and projected it on a wall for the world to see.

"I put myself in an awkward position. But I have a long history of trying to ethically and delicately negotiate my way into this."

Noland: You put yourself in an awkward position, perhaps. But in reading this article, you come out all right. You have a piece up at the museum. You have your job at Duke. I seem like an overwrought woman who couldn't understand the meaning of art. According to this journalist, no one involved in this controversy could identify with my position. No one could understand why I might be hurting. The museum couldn't imagine why I would be upset. You feel awkward and distressed, but you believe your work is "valid."

You're in an awkward position, but mine is compromised.

"We're being watched."

Not "we," Noland. You're doing the watching. You're a peeping tom, a voyeur, a creep who videoed me and called it art.

———

IN THE INTERVIEW, Noland said, "I'm interested in what people are ceding by constantly using devices that allow them to be charted assiduously by Facebook, marketers, retailers, the government."

Recently, I gave a workshop at a conference on the digital world and how we engage with it. Quite literally, the theme of the conference was our digital presence, and how much we yield, or can control. During our discussion, things often felt fairly nihilistic, depressing even. In any event, we worked together to learn what we could about the digital landscape and surveillance, and while I was there, with this chapter already in progress on my laptop, I thought about what a rookie William Noland is with his baby-boomer video camera.

At registration for the conference, you could select one of two different colors for your name tag lanyard: black or red. A red lanyard indicated that you did not wish to be photographed or videoed for any of the conference media, either by the official photographers or by the attendees. I selected a red lanyard.

And then I thought about what it meant to have a code of conduct—at a conference about the digital, at a conference about how much is out of our control on the internet—that gives attendees control over whether they are photographed. To have a code of conduct that forbids photography without attendees' consent. How easy was it to put in place such a code of conduct, to go beyond what is merely legal? How simple was it to make me, and others like me, feel safe?

Although it is legal to do so—to photograph a person in a public place—this conference's code of conduct created a place in which doing so was a violation. A violation of trust, a violation of a person's bodily autonomy.

What the conference recognized was something that we all can feel: Although it might be legal, it is wrong.

But what about the selfie in Times Square that accidentally captures a tourist behind you? We don't want to give that tourist grounds to sue, right?

As a law professor, I can assure you that the law is capable of recognizing a distinction between that tourist accidentally captured in the background of a selfie and Noland pointing his camera at my face and then projecting it on the wall of a museum three feet tall and five feet wide in order to further his career. Those two things are materially different.

WHEN I KNEW I had to write this chapter, I considered writing it at Caffe Driade, the coffee shop where Noland filmed me for Dream Rooms. After seeing the installation years ago, I've never returned there. Perhaps it is unreasonable of me to also blame the cafe for what Noland did, but I can't help but think that they must have known what he was doing. How could they not? The space is so tiny. The tables so small, so intimate. Knowing Noland and Dream Rooms as well as I do now, I know that's why he picked the spot—the closeness, the intimacy.

When I was an undergraduate, my friends and I used to go there because it felt exotic. We were driving to Chapel Hill from Durham where I went to college, and we parked in the gravel lot deep among the trees, and we'd enter the small, low-ceilinged building, with its Italian name, tucked back far from Franklin Street, and we'd order Italian coffees. We'd read books and write in our notebooks.

I have good memories of those times.

In the tiny building, you can go and sit near others who are, like you, concentrating on their thoughts, their work, their reading or writing or calculations (not lost in the Matrix or whatever nonsense Noland wanted to prove). No, we worked side-by-side at those small, metal-topped tables, trusting each other to watch our stuff while we ran to the bathroom or ordered more coffee, the quiet buzz of the space creating the white noise we needed to concentrate. We trusted. I was able to trust.

But not anymore.

I know Noland isn't there with his video camera (or is he?). But every time I slow my car, climbing the hill up Franklin Street, I can't make myself pull off the road onto that gravel drive. *Did they know?* I wonder. *Were they complicit?* And then the atavistic part of me also has its say —my hands clench on the steering wheel, and my heart beats faster. That small space is no longer safe. I press down on the accelerator and pass by the turnoff, past the small building tucked into the trees, and climb the hill too fast, perhaps. Or perhaps just fast enough.

PART II. THE PUBLIC

9

HOW TO WRITE PUBLICLY ABOUT RAPE

If you want to write publicly about sexual assault, harassment, and rape, then you have to do so deliberately. You have to take some crucial matters into account.

First, and always: You have to take care of yourself.

You can count on no editor to take care of you. Editors will want your stories. But most editors will not take into consideration the harm that making your stories public will cause you. That harm is up to you to consider, and to balance against the good that telling your stories will do.

How do you strike that balance? Here's my advice.

If you want to write publicly about sexual assault, harassment, and rape, you need to keep two things in mind: who you are, and what you need.

I learned the hard way that when I write about sexual assault, harassment, and rape, I have to take care of myself. I didn't train for this work—I'm not sure you can. And no one mentored me. I didn't have a sexual assault writing group. (I do now.) I don't want you to make these mistakes; allow me to help.

Who You Are: Expert or Survivor or Both?

For over ten years, I worked as a full-time professor of writing and of law. I now teach law part-time, and my full-time job is as a professional writer and editor. One of the things I write publicly about is law—especially how the law intersects with sexual assault, harassment, and rape. Sometimes when I write about rape, I write about my personal experience as a rape survivor. Sometimes I don't, preferring to keep my experience as a survivor out of the story and to keep the focus on my legal expertise instead.

The point is, these choices I make about who I am when I write a piece are deliberate. If you want to write publicly about sexual assault, harassment, and rape, then you will have to make choices about who you are as well. But when I first started writing, I didn't understand that I had control over how much of my identity I could put on the page. I thought I had to be a survivor all of the time.

I'm a rape survivor, but I'm also a legal expert on rape. Some media outlets you write for (editors) and some journalists who interview you will want you to be one or the other, but not both. They're wrong. You can be both. You can be a survivor who is also an expert. Your expertise doesn't only derive from being a survivor, and being a survivor doesn't negate your expertise in other areas.

Once, I was a media expert for a reporter doing a piece on campus rape. Remember: I'm a law professor, an attorney, and a legal expert in addition to being a survivor.

But when the piece came out, I was simply "survivor Katie Pryal." None of my expert authority made it into the piece. That wasn't okay, and the interview still bothers me to this day. At the time, I did nothing about the misidentification. I should have. You have the right to call the reporter and demand a correction, which is what I should have done. I should have been referred to as "survivor and legal expert Katie Pryal." That's who I am: I am both things.

You can also choose to not come out as a survivor at all. Sexual assault survivors are under incredible pressure to both keep our assaults secret and to talk about them.

We're pressured to share our stories, especially right now in our era of #MeToo. But at the same time, we are pressured to keep our stories secret for a host of other reasons: shame, embarrassment, or even the fear that no one will believe us.

Then, if you want to write about sexual assault, you might feel like you have to hide your experience as a survivor in order to maintain your credibility as an expert. Can I be an impartial legal expert on sexual assault law if I'm also a rape survivor? Who would believe it?

Of course, one can question whether there is such a thing as an impartial legal expert, but news outlets seem to think they exist, and they seem to think that being a survivor makes a person incapable of understanding how the law works. Sometimes, when I write about rape, I never mention that I'm a survivor at all.

So, beware: editors your write for and journalists who interview you will try to shoehorn you into either "expert" or "survivor." Do what you feel is necessary—be an expert, or a survivor, or both—and don't feel ashamed about what you choose to hide or reveal.

When you write about sexual assault, harassment, and rape, editors can be your best advocates. But they can also be predators. Never forget that your story belongs to you. I've written personal essays for different outlets, and then pulled those essays (even from big outlets!) because the editor wanted me to write things I wasn't willing to. One editor told me I wasn't sharing enough—wasn't digging deeply enough—when I was writing about something traumatic. You need to be able to tell when an editor is correct, and when an editor just wants more of your guts to get more clicks for their site. You need to learn how to keep yourself safe by setting good boundaries. One way is to create a network of writing friends, people you can run editorial notes by. Double-check—are you being too sensitive? Or is this editor asking too much?

By the way: if you feel like the editor is asking too much, then the editor is asking too much.

Similarly, never forget that you are more than your story of survival. You don't have to tell your story of your rape to have a valid story to tell about rape. Like I said above, you can be an expert without revealing that you're a survivor. Forming a good community means finding editors that don't exploit you. Editors will want you to dump your entire soul on the internet for twenty-five dollars. Don't do that. You have a story to tell? Tell it your way, on your terms. There will be an outlet that will fit you better.

Find editors who understand that the story of sexual assault doesn't fit into a single, neat narrative structure of redemption or survival, no matter how much readers may want it to. Your story is your story. It doesn't have to make sense to everyone.

Good editors understand that.

What You Need: Safety, Care, and Community

The writing work I do is important, but it isn't easy. I write about rape because I believe, strongly, that writing about difficult things for the public can change the world for the better. If I didn't believe that the work I'm doing is causing positive change, then I wouldn't do it. I wouldn't be able to do it. It's too hard to do for no good reason.

If you want to write publicly about really hard things, then you need to know why you are writing them. Writing for personal glory isn't good enough. For starters, there isn't any glory. And there certainly isn't any money. You have to believe that the work you are doing matters and that you are making the world a better place. If you doubt yourself, you will stop. And you should. I had to learn on my own that writing will cause backlash. So listen to me now: Writing about sexual assault, harassment, and rape will cause backlash.

Also: I had to learn that there would be spikes of interest in my work, and long lulls of disinterest. I had to learn that spikes and lulls are normal, and not a reflection on my work as a writer. I had to learn to keep writing even through the disinterest. I had to learn to expand my areas of expertise. I had form relationships with other writers.

One of the first pieces I ever wrote for the public was about rape. It appeared in a fabulous online magazine named *The Toast*, a magazine that did a lot to make the world a better place before it closed in 2016. The article I wrote, published in 2014, detailed my experience reporting being raped to a university's Title IX office. (You can read the story in Chapter 3.)

To write the piece, I went through the entire rape reporting process, from figuring out whom to call to report, how to make an appointment, how to find parking, and where to find the Title IX office. There was the waiting—so much waiting—and the uncomfortable meeting with the Title IX representative during which I finally reported the story of being raped in graduate school—years after it happened.

I documented every detail of the reporting process, and then wrote a long-form essay about the experience. I was, in a way, a participant-observer. As an insider to higher education—a professor at the time—I had a unique perspective on reporting being raped. In fact, the entire time I went through the reporting process, the people I ran into along the way kept asking me, "And ... you're a professor?" as if such a thing were unbelievable. Perhaps it was, but I know I couldn't possibly be the only one with this experience. As a professor, writing about my personal experience of sexual assault and reporting it gave the "typical" campus assault story a different angle. That angle made the story I wrote more interesting. (When you write, as you will learn, you will have to have an angle.)

After I published the piece, I suddenly had a voice in the campus rape movement. I received emails of support from readers who found the story an important addition to the literature on campus rape and Title IX. But I wasn't prepared to be a part of a movement. I received a phone call from a person I'd known a decade before, with whom I'd lost touch. She'd become a well-known activist in the campus rape movement. As I was stepping away from academia to write full time, she was emerging as an activist leader. She introduced me to others like her, and I made friends and connections.

I realized, quickly, how important it was for me to have these friends—because, after I published the piece, I made other people angry. Some people on my campus were angry. They thought I'd betrayed our Title IX office by writing about my experience, as though a Title IX office can be betrayed. Others accused me of being spoiled and ungrateful. Others questioned the truthfulness of my rape in the first place. (Of course they did. They always do.)

I was also unprepared for the experience of writing the piece itself. The day I reported my rape to the Title IX office, I drove directly from the office to my sister's house and crawled onto her bed. I told her what had happened, and then I proceeded to shake with a panic reaction for the rest of the day and into the evening. I did my best to hide my physical upset from my children. In short: I hadn't been prepared for what reporting rape, even years later, would be like. I'd thought it would be (relatively) easy. It wasn't. Not at all.

Never underestimate how hard it is to write about sexual assault, harassment, and rape. I'm working hard to stop underestimating how hard this work is. If you are going to write publicly about sexual assault, even if you aren't writing about your own sexual assault, you need to be prepared for the traumatic effects of your subject matter. Writing about trauma causes trauma, every time. You need to plan for it. Build in time for recovery. After you research. After you write a draft. After you file a story. And, especially, on the day the story is published.

When the story hits, you might need space—time away from others while you manage your involuntary reactions to having your words about sexual assault, harassment, and rape published for the world to see. You also need space to manage the reactions you will receive from others, both positive and negative. Whether you are writing about sexual assault as a survivor or not, you will be harassed for your writing. You will need a supportive community both on the internet and in real life. You will need to use social media because, if you are writing for public venues, they will expect you to publicize your work on social media. But if you are on Twitter and you are a woman, you will likely be harassed. It is a given. A community makes it easier to weather and manage the harassment. We help one another out. We learn from one another.

In short: never underestimate the toll that this work can take. Build in time for yourself. If you have to keep working on your regular job on those days, build in more breaks, and don't schedule anything hard. Cut yourself a lot of slack. Be gentle with yourself. When you write about sexual assault, harassment, and rape, you are changing the world, and that's never easy.

10

WHY KESHA LOST

I wrote the piece that is the heart of this chapter in February of 2016, when triple-platinum-selling pop-recording artist Kesha sued for an injunction to stop Sony from forcing her to release records under its label, Kemosabe Records, and from working with the label's founder, a record producer who goes by "Dr. Luke."

Kesha lost her motion for an injunction—and her story captured national attention. A major recording artist's conflict with her label is newsworthy, perhaps, but Kesha's was particularly newsworthy because she alleged sexual abuse at the hands of Dr. Luke. Dr. Luke was a powerful man many years her senior. He exerted massive control over many aspects of her life, not only her career. And she alleged he raped her.

In April of 2016, the judge dismissed all of Kesha's abuse claims against Dr. Luke. However, by April of 2017, Dr. Luke no longer worked for Sony, and he was no longer CEO of Kemosabe Records, the label he founded, for which he produced massive hits for major names in pop music. Dr. Luke, it seems, has withered away to nothing.

But Kesha has not withered away. In August of 2017, nearly five years after the release of her second album, Kesha finally released her third album. She released it under Kemosabe Records, but not with the help of Dr. Luke. The album debuted at number one on the Billboard charts. In October of 2017, she was on the cover of *Rolling Stone* magazine.

I'm not sure what first made me want to write about Kesha. Sure, I'm an activist who writes about sexual assault and how a man's power to control a woman's body so often means he has the power to control her career—and vice-versa. But I know that after I read, just a little, about this case, I became captivated by Kesha Rose Sebert, the young girl, the music geek from Nashville, whose mom wrote songs for Dolly Parton, who wanted to sing songs and make records, and who ended up in the hands of, at best, a megalomaniac, and at worst, an abuser and rapist.

I saw the photographs of her weeping in the courtroom. And I saw her little-girl signatures on the contracts. And I realized that I needed to know more about her story.

February 2016

Last Friday, a judge ruled that she wouldn't release pop singer Kesha from her recording contract with a producer who allegedly raped and abused her for a decade. Support has poured out from many other pop singers including Lady Gaga (whose fiery deposition in this case was recently unsealed), Janelle Monae, and most recently Taylor Swift, who donated $250,000 to Kesha's legal battle.

When I first heard about the February 2016 Kesha injunction ruling, the lawyer in me immediately thought, "How old was Kesha when she signed the original deal?"

To find out, I went docket-diving, pulling the supporting documents from the case, including the original contract signed between Kesha and her producer back in 2005. Kesha Rose Sebert was born March 1, 1987. Eleven years ago, when she signed her record deal with super-producer Lukasz "Dr. Luke" Gottwald, she was barely eighteen. On the contract, her signature has the scrawl of a high schooler, someone still unaccustomed to signing her name on a regular basis.

Had Kesha signed the contract while she was still a minor, the contract would have been voidable. But she was 18, legally old enough to sign away her first six albums to a man she barely knew, a man she alleges turned out to be a monster. And the recent ruling protected only the alleged monster and his corporate masters, not Kesha.

As a lawyer, I can understand the technical reasons why the judge ruled as she did. But as a woman, a feminist, and yes, a lawyer, I think she got it wrong.

To understand the ruling, and why it is wrong, we have to understand who Dr. Luke is, and the power he exerts in the recording industry.

Long before Kesha became Ke$ha, Gottwald, along with his then-mentor Max Martin, wrote and produced megahits such as Kelly Clarkson's "Since U Been Gone" (2004) and Katy Perry's "Kissed a Girl" (2008). In 2009, Gottwald produced his first solo #1 hit, "Right Round" by Flo Rida.

Kesha provided an unpaid hook for the song. That hook helped launch Kesha's career even though she never made a penny off of it.

When Kesha was seventeen and living on a prayer in Los Angeles, Gottwald was thirty-two, nearly twice her age, and well on his way to becoming one of the most successful pop music producers in history. According to *Billboard Magazine*, Gottwald "has garnered 21 top 40 Hot 100 singles, becoming the producer with the third most such hits in the history of the Billboard charts."

In other words, he is a hitmaker. And is very, very valuable to Sony Records. Way more valuable, one could argue, than Kesha. She's just another nearly-former pop star who can be replaced by the endless stream of bright young women who are used, devalued, and eventually destroyed by the entertainment industry—in a perfectly legal fashion.

Gottwald instigated the relationship with Kesha after hearing a demo tape that got passed along to him. In a 2010 *Billboard Magazine* cover story on Kesha, the reporter marvels at Gottwald's discovery of Kesha. When Gottwald first heard Kesha's demo, she was still a goofy high schooler. Gottwald called her home in Nashville out of the blue. "Eventually he got Ke$ha on the phone, and then to a meeting in New York. Ke$ha left [high school] behind and moved to Los Angeles."

She was seventeen. And by eighteen she had signed with Gottwald. She alleges in her complaint that Gottwald first sexually assaulted her shortly after her eighteenth birthday and threatened her about ever exposing his abusive behavior.

He threatened that if she ever mentioned the rape to

anyone, he would shut her career down, take away all her publishing and recording rights, and otherwise destroy not only her life but her entire family's lives as well. He also threatened her and her family's physical safety. Kesha wholly believed that Dr. Luke had the power and money to carry out his threats; she therefore never dared talk about, let alone report, what Dr. Luke had done to her.

After Kesha brought her lawsuit and looped in Sony as a defendant, Sony responded: "Sebert cannot have it both ways...She cannot claim that Gottwald intimidated her into silence, then—as an apparent afterthought—seek to hold Sony...liable for failing to act on conduct that she did not report."

Her legal claim is that Sony failed to act on knowledge that Gottwald was abusive toward women he worked with, including Kesha. My question is this: Is Kesha's reporting of the alleged abusive behavior the only way that Sony could have discovered it? Why does the weight seem to sit only on a single woman's shoulders to bring down a serial abuser?

Harvey Weinstein. Bill Cosby. A code of silence protects men in power against not only the direct victims of their (alleged) abuse, but also against the bystander witnesses of abuse. In each of these other cases, we ask ourselves, *Why did everyone else keep silent for so long? Why do bystanders enable serial abusers and rapists to continue to rape and abuse?*

And our legal system, when it remains willfully ignorant of the power dynamics of the music industry—as the judge in Kesha's case was—enables them as well.

If Kesha's allegations are true, then the following are likely true as well: Bystanders knew about her abuse at

Gottwald's hands. And Gottwald abused other young women. What will it take to believe Kesha? A line of women as long as Weinstein's? Cosby's?

Kesha is hardly the first artist to sue to be released from a multi-record contract. George Michael, for example, immediately comes to mind. Usually, these lawsuits arise because of artistic differences. But I think Kesha's case is unprecedented—because she is not suing because of artistic differences. She is suing because she alleges that her producer is a serial rapist and abuser and that her label, Sony, props him up.

And on February 19, 2016, a New York state trial judge, Shirley Werner Kornreich, sided with the producer and corporation and stated that Kesha had no grounds for a preliminary injunction.

I would argue that Kesha has no grounds that are visible to the court because what she's arguing is brand new. Her case has no precedent in entertainment litigation as far as I can tell. An analogy that might make sense is an unsafe workplace lawsuit against a factory that has a toxic gas leak.

Toxicity is an apt metaphor. Women in the entertainment industry are not supposed to stand up to toxic abusers, whether those abusers are individual men or corporations. As Madeleine Davies at *Jezebel* put it in an article on Kesha, corporations (and men) are in much better legal positions than those of us who have "been legally cursed with female bodies and female voices, which are meant to be soft and agreeable." Kesha, whether because she'd had enough or because she'd reached a point where she felt confident enough to do so, ceased being soft and agreeable.

So why did Kesha lose her motion for preliminary injunction? First, a bit about where the lawsuit stood at the time of the injunction ruling. In October 2014, Kesha filed a civil lawsuit against Gottwald, his record label, and the parent company Sony, alleging many things, including sexual abuse by Gottwald. While this civil lawsuit has been moving through the courts, she's been unable to have anything to do with her music, her brand—anything "Ke$ha"—without working with the very people she's suing—her alleged rapist and Sony.

In September 2015, Kesha filed a motion for a preliminary injunction that would allow her to resume making music and to stop Gottwald and Sony from enforcing the exclusivity contracts she'd signed with them.

In most jurisdictions (including New York), courts will allow preliminary injunctions—which are temporary—so long as two things are true: the requesting party is likely to win the underlying lawsuit and the party will suffer "irreparable harm" if the injunction isn't granted. Kesha's lawyer provided more than adequate proof of irreparable harm to her career should Kesha's career continue to stall.

So why didn't Judge Kornreich grant the preliminary injunction?

On the most basic level, Kesha lost because Judge Kornreich ruled Kesha was not going to suffer irreparable harm: "There has been no showing of irreparable harm. She's being given opportunity to record." The judge is referring to the fact that Gottwald and Sony have agreed to allow Kesha to record under Sony with a producer other than Gottwald.

If you're Kesha, though, you want the ability to choose to work with a producer who can help you succeed as you have been, whether that producer is at Sony, or at any other recording company. You don't want Sony's second-string producer when you've had their star your whole career. You want—you deserve—another star. That's what irreparable harm means. You get the same success you've had all along, before you were (allegedly) wrecked by an abuser.

Indeed, Kesha's lawyer argued that such a promise was "illusory," given that Gottwald is the hitmaker that Sony is invested in, and that not working with Gottwald would essentially mean Kesha was being set up to fail. The judge refused to believe the argument: "You're asking me to assume an entity like Sony, who are in a competitive position, will not want to make money on their investment."

Their "investment": the judge, of course, was talking about Kesha herself. At that point, anyone in the courtroom should have known Kesha was going to lose. By calling her an "investment," the judge reduced Kesha, a person, to a corporate asset.

As a lawyer, I know that Judge Kornreich worked well within the boundaries of existing law. If Kesha can indeed record music, in the eyes of the law, any harm she's suffered over the past few years has been self-inflicted. She chose to stop making music.

Put another way, of course, Kesha chose to stop making music with her alleged rapist and her alleged rapist's company. But for the purposes of the hearing in front of this judge, her allegations of suffering just did not matter.

But Judge Kornreich didn't stop once she pointed out the lack of irreparable harm to Kesha, the point at which Kesha lost the motion. No—the judge also discussed the merits of the underlying rape allegations. And she cast serious doubt on them, by pointing out the lack of medical evidence such as hospital records. But arguably, a contract injunction hearing wasn't the time for such doubting. The judge had already decided that Kesha would lose the injunction—she didn't have to question her credibility as a rape survivor too. That's Gottwald's attorney's job.

Judge Kornreich also called Kesha's injunction request an "extraordinary" one. But Kesha's request was for a preliminary—that is, temporary—injunction, not a permanent one. Furthermore, if the judge had granted the preliminary injunction, Kesha would have had to put money into a court fund (called a "bond") to reimburse Sony and Gottwald for any losses they might suffer due to the injunction should they end up winning the underlying case.

So I disagree with Judge Kornreich. A preliminary injunction is precisely the tool a judge can use in an unprecedented case like Kesha's. It's just the tool you can use to protect a vulnerable person against a behemoth corporation and an alleged predator. The corporate interests would be protected by the bond, and Kesha would be protected by the injunction.

But Judge Kornreich didn't use this tool to temporarily protect Kesha. Instead, she followed her "instinct." She stated, "My instinct is to do the commercially reasonable thing."

How did she decide what was "commercially reasonable"? She looked at the contract and drew some conclusions: "You're asking the court...to decimate a contract which was heavily negotiated and signed by two parties in an industry where these kinds of contacts are typical."

With her words, the judge revealed her presumption: that an 18-year-old Kesha Rose Sebert and a hitmaker nearly twice her age were negotiating equitably back in 2005.

No, Judge Kornreich. They were not.

She stated that theirs was a contract "typical" to the "industry."

Here I agree with Judge Kornreich. This kind of contract is, indeed, typical. It is typical for there to be such a vast power differential in the music industry between a producer and a new artist. And, as the recent allegations against powerful men in entertainment have shown, it is typical for there to be the kind of abuse Kesha alleges, too. No one, including Judge Kornreich, should be surprised by the dark underbelly of the entertainment industry.

But our courts don't know what to do about it, at least not yet. And that's a serious problem.

―――――

WHEN I WROTE about Kesha in February of 2016, I didn't know, then, that she would recover, that she would make music again. Revisiting these words now, with the knowledge that she made her best album after escaping Dr. Luke, I feel hope.

I feel hope for all of us who know what it's like to feel as though we've lost everything to an abuser. And for her to have this success while her abuser fades to obscurity?

She's probably above savoring that.

But I'm not.

11

COSBY AND RETHINKING STATUTES OF LIMITATIONS

In August of 2019, as I was finishing up this book, New York State passed the Child Victims Act (CVA), which lengthened its statute of limitations on childhood sexual abuse. Before the CVA, victims had to bring a suit five years after reaching majority—by the age of 23. Now, they have ten years—by the age of 28. Additionally—and notably—they have granted a one-year period during which anyone can bring suit, no matter how much time has passed. Thus, for one year from the signing of the act, there was no statute of limitations on child sexual abuse at all. As this book went to print, this grace period to bring lawsuits was still in effect.

Between the abuse that pervaded the Catholic Church, and the #MeToo movement during which so many women came forward with abuse claims years after the statutes of limitations had expired, debate raged about whether there should be statutes of limitations on crimes at all. I wrote about the issue because I knew that statutes of limitations exist for a reason—a good reason—but at the same time, the statutes should be tailored to the crimes. Perhaps, I thought, the balance of interests needed to be reexamined.

February 2016

As I watched the multiple allegations of rape against Bill Cosby accumulate, I did what every legal geek would do: I checked the statutes of limitations. Because the women who were accusing Cosby of sexual assault hailed from various jurisdictions, and because statutes vary depending on the state, I knew that geography would play a deciding factor in whether Cosby was tried in the court of public opinion, or in a court of law. When charges were finally brought against Cosby in Pennsylvania in December of 2015, for a crime first reported in 2004, the prosecutors who brought charges squeaked in just under the twelve-year mark of the state's statute.

In North Carolina, where I live, there is no statute of limitations for felonies at all—including sexual assault. North Carolina is one of sixteen states that allow a sexual assault survivor to report the crime solely on the survivor's timeline, rather than the timeline of the statutory code. In criminal law, statutes of limitation have one purpose: to limit the amount of time a victim has to come forward and for the state to bring charges. Once the statute has expired, the state no longer possesses jurisdiction over the crime. Expiration of the statute has no bearing on an alleged perpetrator's innocence, of course.

The issue here—with the Cosby case in particular—is that sexual assault and sex-based violence cases are materially different than other types of crimes when it comes to reporting. Research shows that it's common for a considerable amount of time to elapse before a victim comes forward.

In light of this prosecution against Cosby—and the marked lack of prosecution for the other alleged crimes he committed—attorney and journalist Jill Filipovic argued that the remaining U.S. states should get rid of their statutes of limitations for sexual assault. Writing in the *New York Times*, Filipovic argued that the singular nature of the crime of sexual assault—including the known reticence of its survivors, the foot-dragging of police and prosecutors, and the backlog of rape kits—is reason enough to change the law.

As a former lawyer, I know Filipovic has a point, especially when you consider the inconsistent nature of statutes of limitations nationwide. Why, for example, does Colorado reserve the right to prosecute an alleged forger forever, but not an alleged rapist of an adult woman? Why do rape victims have their entire lives to seek justice in Texas, but only a decade in California? How do we weigh the public policy reasons for having statutes of limitations against the very real difficulties faced by many sexual assault survivors?

This isn't to say statutes of limitations serve no purpose. Richard E. Myers is a former defense attorney, former federal prosecutor, and current professor at the University of North Carolina School of Law. Myers explains the practical, and socially beneficial, reasons why statutes exist for other crimes. For one thing, the quicker the trial, the more (potentially) accurate the prosecution can be. "The prosecution wants a [statute of limitations] because it encourages prompt action," he says. "We want to encourage the investigators to act and witnesses to come forward in a timely fashion."

The second reason concerns fairness. "If you allow a case to get really old, it skews heavily in the prosecution's favor," Myers tells me. "The defense is more likely to lose witnesses than the prosecution." The third reason also relates to fairness, but with a social justice tilt: "We believe in fresh starts. We believe in people rehabilitating. Going back twenty years [to prosecute a crime] ... feels unfair to many people. People should be judged on the basis of who they are now."

But what about sexual assault or sex-based crimes? Is there something unique about these crimes that merits lengthening the statutes of limitation, or, as Filipovic argues, scrapping them altogether?

According to Sherry H. Everett, an award-winning domestic violence attorney and adjunct professor at the University of North Carolina School of Law, the answer is yes—there absolutely is.

Sexual assault or abuse victims often take longer to come to terms with their own crimes, a problem rooted in society's longstanding prejudice against rape victims. "A big part of the victimization of women—all kinds of victimization and abuse—includes the perpetrators convincing her that she's not actually a victim, that she's crazy for thinking the perpetrator has done anything wrong," Everett tells me. These feelings often lead victims to wait to report crimes, especially when the perpetrator is not a stranger.

Indeed, in Everett's experience with her clients, women often have trouble asking Everett for help, telling her things like, "I don't know if I need a lawyer. I don't know if I should be in court right now." Everett notes that self-doubt among victims is very common. "I'll get a description of a horrific victimization that a woman has undergone. And her next line is either: 'Did I bring this on myself?' or 'I played a part and we're both wrong,'" she says. "And we're talking about clearly illegal, black-and-white behavior on the part of the perpetrator."

The high degree of self-doubt, coupled with feelings that the victim is somehow also to blame, is somewhat unique to sex-based crimes and sexual violence, according to Everett—and according to research on such crimes.

A longer statute of limitations, according to Everett, "would give community agencies, such as rape crisis centers, time to support victims and get them to a point where they're ready and able—emotional, mentally, financially—to come forward and report a crime." Everett also made the point that many rape victims are "financially dependent on their rapists," and may need time to become financially independent before taking any legal action. In a state with a short statute of limitations on crimes of sexual violence, however, a victim might not have that kind of time.

In the example of Cosby, newly elected district attorney Kevin Steele finally chose to bring charges on a crime that a victim first reported in 2004. Cosby's legal team repeatedly attempted to stall and dismiss the case, but in February 17,

2016, Montgomery County Judge Steven O'Neill ruled that the case should continue to trial. Everett notes that just as in any other crime, a prosecutor can choose not to prosecute. But the limited timeline presented by statutes of limitations can be very disempowering for victims.

Case in point: In 2005, then-District Attorney Bruce L. Castor, Jr., declined to bring charges against Cosby, claiming there was insufficient evidence to prosecute. In that situation, the victim reported a sexual assault crime in a timely fashion. But the justice system dragged its feet for years, nearly allowing the statute of limitations to expire. In a jurisdiction with a shorter statute of limitations, charges might never have been brought.

Ultimately, the problem isn't *only* statutes of limitations. It's that the U.S. legal system still has not wised up to the unique factors that complicate crimes of sexual assault and other forms of sex-based violence. These factors include the status of the victims, who may feel ashamed or may live dependent on their abusers. Then there are the very real dangers posed by poorly trained police, evidence obstacles (including an enormous rape-kit backlog around the country), and doubtful prosecutors. These challenges create a very real barrier between justice and the victims of crimes that generally do not exist when dealing with, say, allegations of auto theft.

We need to have a national conversation about whether rape charges should be treated like murder cases—that is, without the constricting effects of statutes of limitations. And quickly. Because when weighing the legal implications of statutes of limitations against the needs of this particular class of victims, it becomes clear that justice cannot adequately be served under the pressures of a ticking clock—not yet.

In 2018, Bill Cosby was convicted of assaulting Andrea Constand and sentenced to three to ten years in state prison. He appealed his conviction in June of 2019, and his appeal was pending at the time of this printing.

12

HANDLING INSTITUTIONAL ATROCITIES
WHAT WE CAN LEARN FROM U.S. GYMNASTICS

It seems that every few months there's another horrifying sexual assault scandal at a university or other institution. The latest, at the time of this printing, is Michigan State University and U.S. Gymnastics' complicity in the abuse Larry Nassar inflicted on athletes at MSU and after he left to join the USA Olympic Gymnastics program. Other stories of institutional atrocities abound: Baylor's football program has, over the years, enabled and covered up sexual violence, and before that, Penn State football enabled rampant child abuse, at the center of which was child abuser assistant coach Jerry Sandusky and what long-time head coach Joe Paterno did and didn't know over the years that Sandusky abused children. The University of Oregon tried to brush a gang rape by three basketball players under the rug, allowing them to play in the National Collegiate Athletic Association tournament and then transfer to other schools before they got in real trouble. Then the school harassed the accuser in unconscionable ways.

If you were a woman, say, and a journalist who covers higher ed and sexual assault (like I do), you might feel like moving to an uninhabited island from sheer exhaustion from the constant *constantness* of these events.

Journalist Jessica Luther, who helped break the story about Baylor University's complicity in the crimes committed by its athletes, has pressed on. Dvora Meyers, a journalist who covers gymnastics, has relentlessly covered Nassar's crimes and trial. The point is, we don't give up. We can't. Someone has to hold these institutions' feet to the fire—because if we don't, they won't do the right thing. They won't feel ashamed and act accordingly.

Jemele Hill, a sports journalist, wrote an article in September of 2017 for *The Undefeated* about MSU, which happens to be her alma mater. It's the place where she started her journalism career. She wrote, "Michigan State needs to wear this shame. The university deserves this humiliation, derision, doubt, discomfort and every unkind word. We need to listen to every word from the victims and absorb all of their anger. They've dealt with this betrayal and violation of their trust for years. Michigan State only has to survive a few news cycles."

Hill even points to comparable situations at other schools: "Michigan State is getting off light compared to the outrage directed at Baylor and Penn State during and in the aftermath of their sexual abuse scandals." But the point she's making is the point that those of us who write about these atrocities are all trying to make—institutions only act in their own self-interest, despite what they may preach in their mission statements: "When protecting institutions, friendships, business partnerships and image become more important than protecting vulnerable people, you get what you deserve."

Every institution facing unbelievable pain that their own failures helped inflict only has one viable path: One of deep apology. Shame. Grief. And if these outpourings turn out to be sincere, healing. But the problem is, colleges and universities are too quick to push the pain under the rug, sacrificing the victims on the altar of public image. And the consequences of doing so are dire.

One could ask (indeed, these questions are asked all the time): how can predators like Nassar, Sandusky, and others have committed their crimes, crimes with such scope and over such a long period of time? The answer is the same for any serial perpetrator (serial rapist cop Daniel Holtzclaw comes to mind): the victims are afraid to come forward, and when they finally do, no one believes them or has urgency to act upon their word. For example, Daniel Holtzclaw deliberately selected women who were poor and had outstanding criminal warrants as his victims—women who were afraid to come forward to report him.

Let me repeat what I just said: perpetrators of sexual assault depend on their victims being afraid to come forward. They depend on their victims being disbelieved and being disregarded. Those three things make sexual assault perpetrators feel invincible. And, for so long, or perhaps forever, perpetrators are invincible. So long as victims are afraid, or disbelieved, or disregarded, perpetrators can rape and abuse with impunity. How can they be stopped?

Institutions can stop them. They can create environments that enable atrocities, or not. The responses of institutions to the Nassars, to the gang rapes, and to the Sanduskys create environments that can either nurture victims or nurture perpetrators. My advice: Don't nurture the perpetrators. Institutions: You have a choice about the message you send—not just to your own constituents, but to the wider world as well.

Here are some words that will let victims know they don't need to be afraid, that they will be believed, that they won't be disregarded:

We have done a horrible thing. We have allowed a horrible thing to happen. The horrible thing was all our fault. We will never, ever allow it to happen again. You are safe here, now. We swear it.

Those words will change the world. It seems so easy. And yet, it isn't easy when your public relations team is telling you that simple words like those above might put you and your institution at risk.

If you're an administrator of an organization like a university or a sports program, and you are reading this column, and you are facing a choice, I beg you.

Say those words.

If you do so, tomorrow, a rape might be reported that otherwise might not have been. And that report might avert another. And just like that, your words might create a culture where a Nassar can never be.

That's why MSU needs to wear its shame. And so should Baylor and Penn State and U.S. Gymnastics and Oregon and every institution that has put its reputation above the welfare of the people it claims to care for.

13

SO MANY BRETT KAVANAUGHS

I went to college with Brett Kavanaugh.

No, not really. Brett Kavanaugh is a lot older than me. Plus, he went to Yale University, and I went to Duke, a mildly less prestigious university many states away.

But, on Duke's campus, I was surrounded by Bretts: by the many wealthy, white men who thought they deserved sex with women both on campus and off. These Bretts were everywhere. And so, unsurprisingly, was campus sexual assault. At Duke, like women did at so many other university campuses that cater to a certain type of wealthy, white man, women had to tolerate the Bretts.

We lived in a Brett Bubble. We had no other option.

Lately, there's a lot of focus on campus sexual assault, which is heartening. Much of the focus is on student-athletes, however, which is less heartening. In fact, one of the biggest campus sexual assault scandals involving Duke centered on its men's lacrosse team, back in 2006. If there is one thing that the Duke lacrosse case does, it is elicit strong opinions. And, one could argue, the Duke lacrosse case isn't about campus rape at all. Weren't the alleged rapists cleared?

In the Duke lacrosse case, there are a few things that happened for certain: Over spring break in 2006, the men's lacrosse team hosted an off-campus, drinking party replete with underage drinking at a house on North Buchanan Avenue, which was located directly across the street from Duke's East Campus. For the party, the men's lacrosse team hired two Black, female dancers to perform at the house. Before the start of spring break, the men's lacrosse coach gave each player a large sum of cash, ostensibly for food over break—$500 each according to one player—which means, say, if 30 of the 47 players were at the house, there might have been $15,000 in cash there. Only one of the players on the team was Black, and the rest of the players were white. The party ended with animosity between the players and the dancers, and at least one lacrosse player called the dancers the n-word as the dancers left.

These are the facts that are not in dispute by anyone involved in the case.

Let's suppose that what I described above is all that happened—no rape or assault. Just this: most of the team's players with thousands of dollars in cash, drinking underage with no legal consequences, believing it was OK to hire two women to come to their house to perform adult dancing and to verbally abuse the dancers as they left.

What kind of bubble do you have to live in to think that that kind of behavior—which according to neighbors in that East Campus neighborhood happened all of the time at the lacrosse house—would yield no negative consequences whatsoever? No arrests, no harassment by police, no loss of future prospects. Nothing.

That's the Brett Bubble.

We saw the Brett Bubble on display during the Kavanaugh hearings, when Brett Kavanaugh showed his angry frustration, like a toddler who had his iPad taken away. He couldn't believe he was being held accountable for his bad behavior in college. He couldn't believe that someone, a woman, was threatening the bubble of nonaccountability he'd been used to his entire life.

I graduated from Duke in 1998—years before the 2006 lacrosse case. But I didn't leave Durham, not really. I lived in the same neighborhood of that off-campus lacrosse house for most of the years I was in law school, and then for years after that, after I met the man I eventually married. I was that house's neighbor. Years after that awful night in 2006, I stood across the street on East Campus and watched the house get demolished after it sat empty, derelict, for years. It fell down like a house of cards.

When I enrolled at Duke in the mid-nineties, I was eighteen years old. I had come from boarding school, which in many ways prepared me for college. I could do my own laundry, manage my meals, and handle time for homework, social life and the like.

In other ways, though, I wasn't ready for Duke at all. My high school didn't have a football team, or any big-time sports, not like Duke does. And Duke's fraternity life shocked me. At Duke, the fraternities are located in dorms on campus. And because the best housing on campus houses fraternities, the participation in fraternities is high—when I was there, participation was roughly 50% for fraternities—and sorority participation was at 60%. That's far higher than the roughly 20% participation in Greek life at the nearby University of North Carolina at Chapel Hill.

Greek life dominated at Duke, and it revolved around alcohol. Drinking was a part of the culture. And attending Duke, for most Duke undergraduates (though not me), was about three things: partying, spending your parents' money (or pretending to if they didn't have it), and making connections so you could get a killer banking job when you graduated or so you could get into medical school. Duke wasn't about learning, but *scoring*—and for the guys, it was about scoring in every sense of the word.

In short, when I was at Duke, I was surrounded by Bretts, and they made Duke a miserable place to be.

I tried to ignore the Bretts, the way one ignores mosquitoes on a camping trip. They don't stop biting, and you don't stop bleeding, but the pain recedes in your mind in its incessant incessantness. I graduated in three years, and I spent the next twenty years tossing requests for my alumni donations into the recycling bin.

But then the Kavanaugh hearings happened, and I had to listen to his excuses, anger and self-righteousness, and so many awful memories came back.

Kavanaugh now has a lifetime judicial appointment, and I'm a lawyer and former law professor. Supreme Court opinions are my Shakespeare. For the rest of my life (not just the life of Justice Kavanaugh), I will be forced to interact with Supreme Court opinions he has authored or co-authored. He is now a permanent fixture in my professional life.

His is a similar situation to Justice Clarence Thomas. I'm

old enough that I watched Professor Anita Hill testify in hearings when Thomas was nominated. I have spent my entire professional life with a known sex abuser on the highest court in the land. And there is nothing we can do about it. What does that teach us about justice? What does it teach our children?

I didn't want those Brett memories back, to be honest. I wanted them to stay gone, like the lacrosse house off of East Campus, flattened by the passage of time and by neglect. But they came back nevertheless.

One Brett at Duke, a guy I met in a poetry seminar, showed up at my on-campus apartment one evening, claiming he'd locked himself out of his place. "No problem," I said, "you can crash here until morning." I thought he was really nice, smart, and sensitive. In the night, he snuck into my bedroom, and I pushed him off of me. The situation was very uncomfortable, and I fell back asleep. He masturbated on my bed while I was asleep and then left. I didn't know he'd done this foul thing until morning, when I discovered the mess he'd left behind. I didn't tell anyone.

Another Brett, a guy I'd met one summer and played sports with, showed up at my apartment to hang out. He was fun and kind, I thought. As the evening wore on, he started crying, begging me to sleep with him. I said "No." He grabbed me and tried to forcibly kiss me. I pushed him off of me. He ran out the door. I avoided him on campus after that. I didn't tell anyone.

I could go on. There were so many Bretts. They were all awful, and they are likely successful now. Duke, and places like Duke, grew Bretts like weeds.

If one of those Bretts who hurt me were nominated for the Supreme Court, what would I do? Would I testify in Congress? Could I be so brave? I hope so. I hope I could speak for all of the other women who've been harmed, to say, "There are other men and women who could do this job, men and women who do not believe that they're better than everyone else, that they can hurt people with no consequences. Let's give them the job, instead."

PART III. ON CAMPUS

14

HOW CAMPUS RAPE CHANGED MENTAL HEALTH PRIVACY FOR ALL

Sometimes what we write changes the world. This chapter tells the story of one of those times—one of the few times that I made a material difference—a difference I could see—with a story I wrote. The first story collected in this chapter struck a chord the brought about real change; the second story collected here recounts some of the ways my writing, and the bravery of the rape survivor at the heart of the story, made a difference in the world.

The first story was wonkish and boring, or so I thought at the time. It concerned FERPA—the Family Educational Rights and Privacy Act. It also concerned an ugly campus rape at the University of Oregon, which is why, when the magazine tweeted out the headline, it caught the eye of an ESPN sportscaster. He shared my story with his social media followers—his *one million* social media followers. After that, my life changed, at least for a while.

Here's how.

Chronicle of Higher Education - March 2015

In January of 2015, a rape survivor sued the University of Oregon for mishandling her sexual-assault case. Through the campus judicial process, the university found the three male students responsible for gang-raping her (not the technical term). They were kicked off the varsity basketball team and eventually out of school. But there is a lot more to the story, including the ways that the university delayed the investigation of the students long enough so that they could finish up their basketball season.

The story is long, and it might destroy your faith in humanity, even if the university did drop its counterclaim against the survivor last week. In that counterclaim, Oregon had accused her of "creating a very real risk that survivors will wrongly be discouraged from reporting sexual assaults."

But I want to focus on only one sliver of this case—one ugly, frightening sliver. I guess we can thank the university's administration for shining some daylight on the legal quirk that I'm about to talk about, because otherwise it might have stayed hidden.

The Oregon administration accessed the rape survivor's therapy records from its counseling center and handed them over to its general counsel's office to help them defend against her lawsuit. They were using her own post-rape therapy records against her.

It was a senior staff therapist in the counseling unit who blew the whistle on the administration's actions. In her public letter, she sounds horrified that the work she thought was protected by medical privilege could be violated in such a fashion.

The university came firing back, arguing that because the rape survivor had asserted a legal claim of emotional distress, Oregon was entitled under, of all things, the Family Educational Rights and Privacy Act to use her medical records to defend against her suit.

When I read the university's defense of its actions, I had to laugh. Medical privacy typically can be breached in a lawsuit setting only when a patient sues a health-care provider for malpractice. In those instances, the medical records become material evidence to determine whether the provider had breached medical standards of care.

In the lawsuit, it appears that the rape survivor has not asserted any claim of malpractice against her therapist. Indeed, her therapist—and the entire department in which the therapist works—is standing up for the rights of the rape survivor.

How in the world could the university claim that it, as a party outside of this therapeutic relationship between the client (the rape survivor) and the therapist, has a right to access her medical records for litigation defense? That goes against everything I ever learned studying law, teaching law, and practicing in the malpractice courtroom.

However, after researching Oregon's argument, I stopped laughing. Because it appears that the university was right. By an education-law loophole, it does have a right to her records under FERPA. And that means everything has to change.

If you are a student and seek counseling at your college's counseling center, your medical records are most likely not protected by the typical medical-privacy laws, otherwise known as the Health Insurance Portability and Accountability Act. Instead, they fall under the aegis of FERPA, just as Oregon said. And compared with HIPPA, FERPA is about as protective as cheesecloth.

When the university accessed the rape survivor's medical records, not even her own therapist knew that the university's actions were probably legal. That's because the education laws and medical laws overlap in confusing ways.

The U.S. Education Department recognized this confusion and put out a frequently-asked-questions sheet on its website (latest update, 2008) to clarify matters. This document contains sections that address the very issue that arose at Oregon.

Now, you may know that FERPA applies to most colleges and universities. What you might not know is that, as the FAQ states, FERPA therefore applies to "the records on students at the campus health clinics of such institutions. These records will be either education records or treatment records under FERPA, both of which are excluded from coverage under the HIPAA Privacy Rule." In plain English, college medical records simply do not count as real medical records, at least for privacy purposes.

Although FERPA provides a slightly different definition for "treatment records" than for "education records," the difference is, shall we say, academic, because the same disclosure rules apply: "[A] school may disclose an eligible student's treatment records for purposes other than the student's treatment provided that the records are disclosed under one of [FERPA's] exceptions to written consent." And one of those exceptions to disclosure with consent? When the student sues the institution.

The university is right, under the law. It can access the therapy records of a rape survivor in order to defend itself against a lawsuit that has nothing to do with therapy malpractice. That is the ugly truth of this case.

What does this ugly truth mean for you, if you are a student, or for your students, if you teach at an institution?

I've spent a lot of time thinking about the stigma and other challenges faced by rape survivors and by people with psychiatric disabilities (that is, mental illness). In other words, about the challenges faced by people who seek counseling.

My advice is simple.

Students: Don't go to your college counseling center to seek therapy. Go to an off-site counseling center. If, God forbid, you've been sexually assaulted, try to find a rape-crisis center. It will have wonderful people to talk to, free of charge. (I know from personal experience.) You simply do not have adequate privacy protections if you go to a college-provided counselor. Sorry. (Or, in the University of Oregon's case, sorry not sorry.)

Instructors: Don't advise your students to seek counseling in the on-campus counseling center. There is no way that, in good conscience, I can ever give that advice again. If you have a student in crisis, help that student find support off campus.

The problem with my advice, of course, is one of money —serious money, in some instances. Many student-health plans will not pay for students to see a counselor who is not at the institution's own counseling center.

In other words, a student's insurance purchased through a college will pay only for a counseling benefit that lacks adequate medical-privacy protection from the very institution that sold the student the insurance. And a student-health plan is all many students can afford.

So for them, stuck between unaffordable therapy in a safe space and free therapy provided by an institution they are unsure they can trust, what then?

The University of Oregon has shown that when administrators are desperate, when they want to use ugly tactics to intimidate a student who is challenging the status quo, they will. And even if Oregon is an outlier, its initial action could very well chill the desire of students to seek support at university counseling centers everywhere.

So my final piece of advice is directed to the U.S. Education Department: Fix this devastating privacy loophole.

DAME Magazine - September 2015

On August 18, Kathleen Styles, the Chief Privacy Officer of the Department of Education (ED) published new guidance for schools about how they should be protecting student medical records under the Family Educational Rights and Privacy Act (FERPA). It's a move that has far-reaching implications for college students, and is also a rare bit of good news in the fight against rape culture that permeates many campuses.

In order to understand the driving forces behind these legal changes, we need to go back to 2014, to the University of Oregon, and revisit one of the more public and more horrific cases of campus rape.

Early last year, on January 8, a campus sexual-assault survivor at the University of Oregon sued the school for mishandling her case. The assault happened in March 2014. The survivor, who is using the name Jane Doe to protect her privacy, reported a gang-rape by three male students to campus authorities and the police. (Content warning: The report contains an extremely violent depiction of sexual assault.) At the end of the 2013-14 school year, the university found the three students "responsible for sexual misconduct" and banned them from campus for up to ten years.

(The police chose not to prosecute, citing low likelihood of conviction. The alleged gang rapists "didn't deny what happened as much as they said the acts that the accuser described were consensual." Now would be a good time to review that police report, and to check your gut.)

So what's the problem? There were many. The University of Oregon waited until after the end of its basketball season to investigate the assault, even though the survivor reported in March. Why? Because the three assailants were on UO's basketball team. To make matters worse, one of the players, Brandon Austin, was recruited from another school, Providence College, where he'd been suspended from the basketball team for sexual assault and banned from campus by the school's disciplinary board (a ban that was overturned by the school's vice-president so he could continue to attend practice with the basketball team).

In her complaint against UO filed in January, Jane Doe

alleged the deliberate delay in investigation, the deliberate recruiting of a player with a known history of sexual assault, and, most importantly for our purposes here, a violation of her medical privacy.

We learned more about this privacy violation the following month, when employees of the UO student counseling center blew the whistle on one of the most disturbing aspects of the case. Jennifer Morlok, a senior staff therapist at UO's student counseling center claimed in a public letter of concern that, prior to Doe filing her lawsuit, UO employees went through her campus counseling records without Doe's consent.

UO defended the secretive records-grab, arguing that because Doe was claiming emotional distress in her lawsuit, it was entitled to take her counseling records under FERPA. UO argued that it could take the records even before a lawsuit was filed—upon just hearing that there may be a lawsuit filed. Furthermore, they claimed they had a right to do so outside the normal discovery process overseen by our legal system.

At first I couldn't believe the university's gall. UO had used a law—FERPA—that is meant to protect student privacy in order to breach the privacy of a rape survivor. When I learned that such actions were indeed permitted under FERPA, I wrote in a March column, "If you are a student and seek counseling at your college's counseling center, your medical records are most likely not protected by the typical medical-privacy laws, otherwise known as the Health Insurance Portability and Accountability Act (HIPAA). Instead, they fall under the aegis of FERPA, just as Oregon said. And compared with HIPAA, FERPA is about as protective as cheesecloth."

Let's back up a step to understand how FERPA has typically worked when it comes to protecting—or not protecting—student medical records.

FERPA covers the records of students who visit health clinics maintained by schools. These campus medical records are not protected under the regular HIPAA privacy laws. In plain English, for privacy purposes, college medical records simply have not counted as real medical records.

Although FERPA provides a slightly different definition for "treatment records"—those that are created for medical treatment—than for "education records," the difference has been meaningless in action. By definition, treatment records can only be disclosed with the student's written consent. But FERPA has a long list of ways that treatment records lose their special status. If a student takes any of the actions on this long list, their treatment records are "converted" into regular old education records, and education records can be shared without written consent.

Here are some of the actions that a student can take that will convert her treatment records and allow them to be shared without written consent: When a student sues her institution. When a student simply wants to see her own treatment records. In the real world, asking to view your own medical records does not release a medical provider from his or her ethical duty to keep your medical records private. That's because in the real world, your medical records are protected by HIPAA.

The fact that FERPA is all that has kept student medical

records private can have far-reaching consequences, far beyond Jane Doe and UO—even far beyond the privacy of rape survivors. All students' medical privacy has been at risk when student health providers can only give students substandard protections.

An LGBTQ student who seeks counseling about bullying but who isn't out to her family or friends is at risk. A student with a psychiatric disability that carries deep public stigma is at risk. A student who is HIV positive and is suffering depression, a common comorbidity, is at risk. Any of these students might seek counseling or medical care on campus, and their medical records would not be protected by HIPAA. They would only be protected by FERPA. Which, as the UO debacle has shown us, is not much protection at all. And, to make matters worse, the student health providers, the people who are doing the salt-of-the-earth work providing care to the students in need, themselves often don't know that their patients have substandard privacy protections.

In my March column, I recommended that students seek treatment at off-campus medical clinics to protect their privacy. This advice made some people at some schools very angry, but I stood by it. Some university employees argued that, although FERPA allowed the taking of medical records in the way that I described (and, when interviewed, the Department of Education supported my argument), it would be the wrong thing to do, so "students shouldn't worry that counseling centers will share their records without their permission." Students should just trust their schools to do the right thing.

My response: You, school representative for University

ABC, might be a good person. But you don't know what your school's General Counsel's office is going to do when staring down the barrel of a multi-million-dollar lawsuit. You, spokesperson for College XYZ, might be a good person, but you can't make that kind of reassurance when the law explicitly allows school lawyers to grab whatever records they want. You can't just tell students to trust you. That's not fair to students who are in desperate need of help.

Here's where the Department of Education's potential FERPA overhaul becomes really good news.

After accounts of UO's medical records grab went public, a lot of people got angry, including legislators in Washington, D.C. They acted. For example, Suzanne Bonamici (D-Ore.) took leadership on the issue of finding new ways to protect student medical records. Her work and that of others have recently culminated in the new guidance on FERPA meant to provide more protection for students.

To be honest, I'm feeling hopeful. (Fair warning, though: I'm a bit of an optimist.)

The August 18th Department of Education (ED) draft of the Dear Colleague letter and summary blog post are seemingly designed to prevent a UO incident from ever happening again. (A "Dear Colleague Letter" is a publicly issued policy statement by a federal agency that explains existing agency regulations.) ED wants to reassure students that they can be safe in their student health centers. Indeed, ED acknowledged this purpose in the blog post:

> Institutions of higher education have a strong interest in ensuring that students have uncompromised access to the

support they need, without fear that the information they share will be disclosed inappropriately. Providing on-campus access to medical services, including mental health services, can help promote a safe and healthy campus. The practice of sharing a student's sensitive medical records with others not involved in their treatment may discourage the use of medical services provided on campus.

This chilling effect is ED's motivation to act—and it should be schools' motivation as well. Schools should be willing to give up the ability to take students' records outside the proper legal processes in order to give students peace of mind when they access campus services. Students' health should trump schools' ability to win at all costs, and schools should be able to see that. (I warned you I was an optimist.)

And what does ED think should be the model for student privacy? HIPAA:

We think [the HIPAA] standard makes sense, and that FERPA's school official exception should be construed to offer protections that are similar to HIPAA's. We want to set the expectation that, with respect to litigation between institutions of higher education and students, institutions generally should not share student medical records with school attorneys or courts, without a court order or written consent.

This statement suggests that even when a student sues a school, the school must go through the usual legal channels to get its hands on the student's medical records. There is an exception for when a lawsuit is over the actual provision of medical care (e.g., malpractice or failure to pay a bill) but even then, a school "should only disclose those records that are relevant and necessary to the litigation."

Granted, these guidelines are only in "draft" form, and ED is "seeking public input on our draft guidance, as we believe that this input will result in a better product." (Schools have 45 days to comment from the August 18 publication date.) But if these new directives mean what I think they mean, then a gaping privacy hole for students—all students, not just rape survivors—is about to be at least partially filled.

Although the change isn't perfect—I would like to see all medical records actually protected by HIPAA—legal change can be slow. But this change happened in six months. And six months is very, very fast. And we have a campus rape survivor to thank for the change. Jane Doe wrote, in a letter to the editor of the UO campus newspaper, "I know a lot of people are angry. I am angry, too. I am angry with the culture that appears to exist in our athletic department that prioritizes winning over safety of our students."

Had these new FERPA guidelines been in place back in December 2014, UO likely would not have been able to access Jane Doe's medical records without a court order, and certainly not prior to her filing a lawsuit. Since her lawsuit did not put her medical treatment at issue, according to these new guidelines, UO would have had to go through ordinary civil litigation channels to access her medical records. And they would only have had access to those relevant to her legal complaint—not access to whichever ones they felt like taking.

Annie E. Clark, the Executive Director of End Rape on Campus, is supportive of these changes, and credits Jane Doe's lawsuit for helping protect the privacy of all students: "Jane Doe's lawsuit helps all students—not just rape survivors—because it called attention to an existing loophole regarding medical privacy," she said. "As stigmatized as mental health already is, we need to culturally and legally break down the barriers that make people feel unsafe or ashamed to ask for help. And assuring students that their medical privacy will not be breached is one necessary step in the right direction."

Last month, on August 4, UO settled its case with Jane Doe for more than $800,000, a settlement that includes a UO education, an education free of the presence of her assailants since they are banned from campus. Furthermore, part of the settlement includes a promise that "the school will pursue a policy change requiring all transfer applicants to report any disciplinary history at prior schools."

But UO's proposed policy change doesn't stop other schools from recruiting the three former UO basketball players who were found responsible for assaulting Doe. Since leaving UO, Brandon Austin transferred yet again, as have his two teammates. They will all play college basketball elsewhere, on scholarship.

The question of a school's responsibility for a transfer athlete's history of sexual assault has come to the forefront recently given the high-profile case of Samuel Ukwuachu, a Baylor University football player convicted on August 20 of second-degree sexual assault. Ukwuachu had transferred from Boise State to Baylor after being kicked off of his former team for violence against a female student there. Reporting for Texas Monthly, Jessica Luther and Dan Solomon produced an indicting piece showing how complicit college coaches can be in bringing violent students to campus. Some conferences and schools are making moves to make sure that recruits with violent pasts can't transfer to campus. But for Jane Doe, UO's promise to do the same is too little, too late. And even to this optimist, it seems that three men who were found responsible for a heinous sexual assault have escaped meaningful punishment.

15

BANNING COLLEGE ATHLETES FOR SEXUAL VIOLENCE CONVICTIONS IS NOT ENOUGH

Indiana University made the news in 2017 when its faculty athletics committee created a new policy banning the enrollment of prospective student-athletes (both freshman and transfer students) who have a history of sexual or relationship violence. The ban covers athletes who have been convicted of felonies or who have been found responsible in on-campus proceedings of sexual or relationship violence. In its statement about the new rules, IU declared that its "Policy is designed to help protect all members of the Indiana University community." The new policy required the athletics department to "conduct an appropriate inquiry into every prospective student-athlete's background" before recruiting them.

The new policy sounds great, right? It really isn't.

When I first read about Indiana's new rule, my first thought was this: A student can be convicted of felony domestic or sexual battery and still get an athletic scholarship (at any school but Indiana, apparently), but if they're convicted of a minor, nonviolent drug offense, they can't even qualify for federal financial aid, including loans or work-study jobs? That's the worst kind of hypocrisy. But it is also the law under the "Aid Elimination Provision" of the Higher Education Act (HEA) passed in 1998. According to the ACLU and the Department of Education, since it was passed, the provision has barred over 200,000 students from receiving aid. As higher education policy goes, how can we ban a student who got caught with a joint in high school from attending college on the one hand while recruiting a student-athlete who was kicked out of another institution for sexual assault on the other?

But many schools have—systematically and notoriously—looked the other way when recruiting athletes with known histories of sexual violence. The rule at Indiana, and similar rules that have been created recently at other institutions, seek to put a stop to the problem. The Indiana rule looks similar to one the Southeastern Conference (SEC) created in 2015. The SEC rule prevents transfer into the SEC of athletes who were kicked out of their previous sports programs for "serious misconduct," where "serious misconduct" means sexual or relationship violence (but not, say, theft).

Barring the enrollment of student-athletes with felony convictions of sexual or relationship violence or those with findings of responsibility for sexual or relationship violence is a good thing. But the Indiana rule, in particular, is also far more limited than you might think. Much of the recent high-profile transfer-athlete violence that might have prompted such a rule would not have been prevented by these rules at all.

Let's look at a few cases, and compare the effect the

Indiana rule would have had in preventing the violence, that similar rules, such as the SEC rule, would have had.

First, there is the case of Samuel Ukwuachu at Baylor University TX. As Jessica Luther and Dan Solomon reported for *Texas Monthly* ("Silence at Baylor," August 20, 2015), Defensive end Sam Ukwuachu was an All-American who transferred to Baylor in 2013 from Boise State University ID after being kicked off the football team for violence against a female student there. While at Boise State, Ukwuachu was not convicted of a felony, nor did he go through the campus judicial process for his conduct. After transferring to Baylor, Ukwuachu was then convicted of assaulting a female Baylor student.

One of the many scandals of the case was the question of whether the Baylor coaching staff knew of Ukwuachu's violent history at Boise State before recruiting him to campus. Recently, Baylor's football program has come under massive scrutiny for how it has handled sexual assault allegations against its players. The controversy has led to the firing of the head football coach and the resignation of the university's president.

Would Indiana's rule have prevented Ukwuachu's transfer to Indiana? No. Indiana requires conviction of (or a plea to) a felony or a finding of responsibility in a campus judicial proceeding prior to applying to transfer or enroll. And, a conviction or finding of responsibility are both exceedingly rare. Ukwuachu was dismissed from his team, but he was not convicted or officially found responsible. He was not even indicted. In comparison, the SEC's rule only requires *dismissal* from a prior sports program for a student to be banned from transferring. Therefore, had a rule like that been in place at Baylor at the time of Ukwuachu's transfer, the rule would have barred Ukwuachu from joining the Baylor team. (Baylor is in the Big 12 Conference, not the SEC.)

Then there's the basketball team gang rape case at the University of Oregon that came to light in 2014 (and that I discuss in detail in the previous chapter). One of the alleged rapists, Brandon Austin, had transferred to UO after being suspended from his prior basketball team at Providence College (in Rhode Island), also for a sexual assault allegation. Austin transferred away from Providence before he could be found responsible in any campus proceeding, and no criminal charges were brought against him. After the ugly UO rape case came to light, he was dismissed from the team at UO.

Incredibly, Austin's career still didn't end after Oregon.He went on to play on scholarship at Northwest Florida State, a junior college, and he tried out for the NBA. The other two UO players involved in the gang rape case successfully transferred to new Division I programs: the University of Texas El Paso and the University of Houston.

None of the UO players were charged with crimes in Oregon, and they weren't found responsible in UO campus proceedings, either—after being dismissed from the UO basketball team, all three transferred away from UO before campus proceedings could be brought.

It seems, then, that the Indiana rule would do little to prevent violence.

As with Ukwuachu's transfer to Baylor, none of Austin's transfers to or from Oregon or the transfers of the other Oregon players would have been barred by the Indiana rule. After all, even though Austin was twice dismissed from basketball teams for sexual violence, he was never convicted of a felony, and he was never found responsible in a campus proceeding. The same goes for the other two players who transferred from Oregon to new schools. However, their transfers would have been barred by the SEC rule, because the SEC rule takes into consideration a player's dismissal from a previous team, which is often the only punishment a player will ever see. (None of the teams involved here are members of the SEC.)

Yes, let's ban those convicted of sexually violent felonies from receiving athletic scholarships. And let's have a reasonable appeals process as well, so that those students who've made an effort to rehabilitate can have a chance to go to school.

But the Indiana rule is not enough. Crimes of sexual and relationship violence are massively underreported to police. And when they are reported, the conviction rate is egregiously low. Plea deals (the manner in which more than 90% of criminal cases end) often lower felony indictments to misdemeanor convictions. Those of us who work in the field of sexual and relationship violence know felony convictions for rapists and abusers of the victims we advocate for are as rare as unicorns.

Similarly, students rarely report their rapes to campus authorities, and when they do, they rarely seek to file formal complaints. Instead, they seek other protections their schools can provide, such as campus restraining orders or course schedule changes so that they can avoid seeing their assailants.

When we're talking about the secretive world of big-money collegiate sports, a dismissal from a team for sexual or relationship violence speaks loudly. And schools that recruit these players anyway, knowing they have a history of hurting students, are acting irresponsibly. The Indiana rule doesn't go far enough to protect vulnerable students on campus.

But at least Indiana is doing something. Most schools, like Oregon, like the schools that recruited the plays who left Oregon, do nothing at all.

16

WHY WE SHOULD ALL CARE ABOUT FERPA

Recently, I was reading an email conversation on a listserv for colleagues in my field when one particular email caught my eye. A professor had shared an email he'd received from a student by forwarding the student's entire email to the listserv. The forwarded email included not only the student's message to the faculty member, but also the student's email address, full name, and the school the student attended.

I know that people who work with students do stuff like this all the time: we share the goofy or wonderful things students say. "Students say the darnedest things" is basically a favorite pastime of anyone who teaches.

But what this professor did, in forwarding the student's entire email to a listserv of over a thousand people, rather than, say, paraphrasing a student's words, was a clear violation of the Family Educational Rights and Privacy Act (FERPA). And seeing what the professor did made me feel very bad for the student and for my field as a whole. I realize that most people on the listserv probably didn't feel the way that I did about the professor's email. They probably aren't as sensitive to FERPA issues as I am—but they should be. We all should be, whether we work in higher education, or have children who attend school, or want our education system to work the way it should.

This chapter is about why we should all care about violations of FERPA, a set of regulations that many who work in higher education do their best to both abide by and ignore. This chapter is not meant as a substitute for formal FERPA training or advice about the regulations. Instead, I hope to help you understand why FERPA is important for all of us. But this chapter is also about how schools abuse FERPA when under pressure—often in the context of campus rape. FERPA is meant to protect students, not institutions. We need to understand how valuable the law is to our students, and then we need to make sure that institutions don't abuse it.

FERPA Should Be About Protecting Students

FERPA exists to protect both institutions and students (and their families). FERPA is a series of regulations promulgated by the Department of Education that helps clarify how student information should be treated. (It can be found at 20 U.S.C. § 1232g; 34 CFR Part 99.)

Under FERPA, school officials must keep certain student information confidential. That information, for the most part, includes "education records," which are "records that are directly related to a student and that are maintained by an educational agency or institution or a party acting for or on behalf of the agency or institution."

What counts as an education record? Things like "grades, transcripts, class lists, student course schedules… student financial information (at the postsecondary level), and student discipline files." Furthermore, "The information may be recorded in any way, including, but not limited to, handwriting, print, computer media, videotape, audiotape, film, microfilm, microfiche, and e-mail."

Students have a right to request and view their education records, and they have a right to expect school employees to keep their education records private. One big exception to that "education record" rule are records that school employees create just for their own note-taking and that they've shared with no one else. These records are called "sole possession records." Students don't have the right to request and view those.

And parents don't have a right to request and view *anything*. No matter how old a student is, once she enrolls in any postsecondary institution, all rights under FERPA belong to the student, not the parents. That means that even if a student is 17 years old, and even if the parents are paying the tuition, the parents do not have a right to that student's education records.

If a parent calls up a faculty member and asks how his kid is doing in the professor's class, the professor cannot share that information, not without prior written permission from the student to do so.

What's more, the professor can't even *confirm* to a parent that a student is in the class at all. Class rolls and a student's course of study are, after all, education records.

Sometimes, a professor can't even confirm that a student is enrolled at the institution.

Under FERPA, institutions have the right to share what's called "directory information"—such as a student's name, major, and year—with the public without violating a student's privacy. However, a student can opt out of having her directory information made public. If a professor has a student whose directory information is set to private, the professor cannot even acknowledge that she is enrolled at the school.

I've heard some faculty and administrators complain that this "no-acknowledgment" rule is too rigid.

But let's think about why a student might wish to keep her directory information private, and more importantly, from whom. Students on the run from abusers or stalkers, for example, might need that level of privacy. And if you are a young person, and you have been abused, it is likely that your abuser was a parent.

Professors, at the beginning of each semester, receive class rolls. On those class rolls, there are notations that indicate whether a student has opted to have their directory information kept private. I've taught at four different institutions, and every institution has put this information on the class roll. If you're a professor reading this book, let me ask you: Do you check for that notation? And do you respect it? If you don't, then you are not taking care with your students' privacy or safety.

If a parent calls you to "check in on his daughter in your class," and you confirm she is your student, you might have given away a student's location to a person she's in hiding from. Always err on the side of protecting a student's privacy.

Just the other day, I ran into a former student. He's

married now, and he was out with his spouse and new baby. My former student greeted me with a big smile, happy to see me as I was happy to see him. My student introduced me to his spouse. I said hello. We chatted for a bit about the baby, and about what my student has been up to.

Finally, his spouse asked, "How do you know each other?"

I stood in silence. This question, even after all of these years, was not my question to answer.

My former student said, "She was my professor." He specified the course, the year.

After he spoke, I nodded in agreement. But even now, after all of these years, nearly a decade, I respected his confidence. I couldn't know why he might have not wanted our relationship disclosed—and it turned out he didn't mind—but that relationship, that he took a course with me, a particular course at a particular institution at a particular time—was his to disclose, not mine.

The great thing about FERPA is that it protects higher ed workers, too. As a professor, I've developed some kind—but firm—ways of redirecting questions. For example, I'm not allowed to disclose anything to parents. I've run into parents of students at the grocery store—"My daughter is really enjoying your class!" And I simply say, "That's interesting," and smile. I don't confirm that there is a daughter in my class at all. To do so would violate FERPA and the trust my students have put in me.

If a parent asks me directly, "Is my daughter in your class?" I reply, "I'm not sure," and then I recommend that the parent ask the student directly or contact the school registrar. A school registrar is accustomed to fielding these requests. And if you're a parent, know that your child's professor can't answer these questions. We're not being unfriendly—we're protecting your child.

Here's the takeaway: If a student hasn't told her parents that she is enrolled in my class, I do my utmost to protect her privacy, even if she hasn't opted to keep her directory information secret. She might have a reason for the secrecy. And if she has a reason, she might also have a problem, a serious one, and I'm in a position to refer her to people who can help.

Higher ed workers owe it to our students to take care of their privacy. We might never know whose health and well-being our discretion will protect. And parents owe it to us to understand how hard our job is and that we're keeping your children safe. Not every student is facing a dire abuse situation. But all of our students deserve to have their records protected.

Let's return to the listserv email-forward situation that I described at the beginning of this chapter. The professor who forwarded that email violated FERPA because he shared a student's education record with a listserv of over a thousand people. The email counted as an education record because it was correspondence between a professor and a student about that student's education. That is, the professor and the student were emailing about school. And then the professor mocked the student's schoolwork on a listserv, providing all kinds of identifying information in the process. Higher education workers should *never* do that. FERPA means our students are in our care—their information, their privacy, and sometimes their safety.

When Schools Abuse FERPA

But what about the situation at the University Oregon, the story I told in Chapter 17? Here's a summary of what happened, and how it fits into the context here.

At Oregon, the university used FERPA to abuse a student's privacy when the university was staring down the barrel of a multimillion-dollar lawsuit. But the student's bravery, and the bravery of the mental health care worker at the university who blew the whistle on the records grab, changed FERPA to better protect students.

Back in February 2015, I read about a horrifying campus rape. Jane Doe, a female student at the University of Oregon, was suing her school for mishandling her rape case —and for granting admission to her rapist, a transfer student who had been banned from his former campus for sexual assault. At the end of UO's campus investigation, three players on the varsity basketball team had been kicked out of school for gang-raping Jane Doe. But, UO had dragged its feet during the investigation so that the players could finish out the NCAA basketball season. UO eventually settled Jane Doe's case in August 2015 for $800,000, for four years' worth of tuition for Jane Doe, and for a change in policy regarding how they admit transfer students.

Of interest to us here is one specific part of Jane Doe's lawsuit. She accused the school of accessing her medical records—in particular, her mental health records from the student counseling center—before the lawsuit was filed, and thereby violating her privacy. Indeed, the UO administration admitted to taking her medical records in anticipation of her lawsuit, without her permission, and giving them to their general counsel's office to help them prepare a defense. A student mental health care worker at UO blew the whistle on the records transfer. UO claimed their actions were protected by FERPA. And, it turned out, UO was right.

I wrote a column for The Chronicle of Higher Education (CHE) outlining my concerns—how could it be possible that a school could access a student's medical records so easily under FERPA? Why weren't student medical records protected like all other medical records—by the Health Insurance Portability and Accountability Act (HIPAA)? It turned out there was such a thing called "treatment records" under FERPA, which are different from "education records." Treatment records received special protection, and couldn't be shared around campus without the student's written permission. But it also turned out that, under FERPA, it was far too easy to "convert" treatment records into education records, which caused them to lose any special protection they may have had.

For example, FERPA allowed for treatment records to be converted to education records if anyone other than the person providing the treatment looked at the records—including the student herself, or, say, her lawyer. If Jane Doe had asked to see her own treatment records, then her treatment records were no longer treatment records under FERPA. They were education records, and they could be shared around campus without Jane Doe's written permission. Basically, as I wrote for CHE, "compared with HIPAA, FERPA is about as protective as cheesecloth." In the real world, looking at your own medical records doesn't cause them to lose their confidentiality. HIPAA continues to protect them. But in college, under FERPA, it does.

Once Jane Doe's treatment records were converted to education records, UO could access them freely, allowing the school to bypass the protections of the litigation discovery process. Imagine allowing opposing attorneys in a lawsuit to just walk into your doctor's office and take whichever of your records they wanted, relevant to your case or not. That's what happened here: UO just took Jane Doe's records, whichever ones they wanted, with no judicial oversight. FERPA, it turned out, wasn't HIPAA, not even close. And that's what I wrote in my CHE column.

I received a lot of angry responses to my CHE column. There were those who were angry because they thought I'd misread the law (a "you got it wrong" argument; this one was the most common). There were those in the mental health profession who were angry, for some reason, that I had brought the records-grabbing to light. They were very protective of the sanctity of the mental health profession, and they thought I'd violated that sanctity (a "you made us look bad" argument). High-level administrators (all men, by the way) told me that, even though I got the law right, they certainly wouldn't do what UO did (a "just trust us" argument; this one was my favorite). One guy said it didn't matter that FERPA allowed for the records grab because all of the records would have come out in discovery anyway. I guess he doesn't have much respect for judicial oversight and the other protections of the discovery process. I do.

It turns out I had read the law right. Folks from Congress gave me a ring and asked me for advice on how to make FERPA better. I said the answer was simple. Make

FERPA like HIPAA. HIPAA, the medical privacy law that protects your medical records unless you're a college student, should be how FERPA works in practice. Within six months, because of a brave UO student and mental health worker and because of strong leadership in Washington DC, the Department of Education issued new guidance on FERPA. Published in The Dear Colleague Letter on "protecting student medical records," the department advised that "without a court order or written consent, institutions that are involved in litigation with a student should not share student medical records with the institution's attorneys or courts unless the litigation in question relates directly to the medical treatment itself or the payment for that treatment, and even then disclose only those records that are relevant and necessary to the litigation"—not all of them. (A "Dear Colleague Letter" is a publicly issued policy statement by a federal agency that explains existing agency regulations.)

If a school wants medical records for any other kind of litigation—such as the kind in Jane Doe's case—then "the school should not access the student's treatment records without first obtaining a court order or consent."

This new guidance brings FERPA more in line with HIPAA, protecting all students from administrative overreach. The bravery of Jane Doe and of the UO mental health care worker who blew the whistle on the records grab, and the strong leadership and quick action in Congress, has led to stronger protection of student medical records on campus. Their important work has ensured that students who are at their most vulnerable can feel safe asking for help.

Another Dark Side of FERPA

The painful story from Oregon had a positive effect on policy; FERPA now protects students' medical privacy better than it did before. But institutions abuse FERPA in another, unexpected way: to unethically block access to information that is strongly in the public interest—and, incidentally, not protected by FERPA.

Unfortunately, this unethical information-blocking also often arises in the context of campus rape. Here's an example.

In September 2016, the campus newspaper of the University of North Carolina at Chapel Hill, *The Daily Tar Heel*, formally requested specific records relating to campus sexual assault cases. According to the paper, "The request specifically asked for all records of people found responsible for rape, sexual assault or misconduct by University entities." The university refused to meet the request, citing FERPA.

In response to UNC's refusal to release the records, the newspaper filed an official public records request under North Carolina law. (This request was joined by other media organizations.) In response to the public records request, the university's vice chancellor of communications stated that "UNC is firmly committed to FERPA regulations" and that "Carolina has a profound responsibility to protect and vigorously defend the privacy of sexual assault victims and all students, including witnesses, who may be involved in a campus Title IX process."

Let's take a look at the issues at play here. On the one

hand, the university has declared it must use FERPA to protect assault victims and witnesses, and therefore it cannot release the records of assault proceedings. That seems like a legitimate reason to withhold records, right? To protect the privacy of those involved in these sensitive cases?

But let's remember—the newspaper only requested the records of the proceedings in which the accused was found responsible for wrongdoing, and it appears that it only requested the names of those found responsible, not the names of the victims or witnesses. The stated purpose of the records request is to hold the university accountable for investigating and punishing campus rape. The newspaper stated that it doesn't even know if records of this kind even exist. It doesn't know if any students at all have been found responsible for wrongdoing of this kind.

It seems that no one outside of the university administration has information about anything regarding these issues—and that's the problem.

According to the National Women's Law Center (NWLC), the law on this issue is clear. FERPA allows schools to disclose "the final results of any college disciplinary proceeding for a violent crime or sex offense that concludes the accused broke a school rule or policy to a third party. Examples of third parties include witnesses, student groups, or reporters." Thus, under the law, the initial records request by *The Daily Tar Heel* was not barred by FERPA, as the paper only requested results of proceedings in which a student was found responsible for wrongdoing, and the request was made by a reporter.

Furthermore, according to the NWLC, the school can

only disclose the names of other involved students—such as the victim or witnesses—if they consent in writing. It appears that the University of North Carolina has no FERPA-based reason to withhold the requested records from the media, and they are quite capable of releasing the records without releasing the names of victims or witnesses. They just don't want to release the records.

Why not? According to attorney Frank LaMonte, executive director of the Student Press Law Center, although FERPA was "intended to protect only the confidentiality of 'education records,' the law has become a catchall excuse for educational institutions to avoid accountability."

In other words, UNC, like all universities, has a strong interest in keeping the results of student conduct hearings private. What if, in the years the records were requested, not a single student was found responsible for misconduct? What if, during those years, students were found responsible, but their punishments were so light that the university would be embarrassed should the punishments come to light? What if high-profile students, such as athletes, were involved, and they were allowed to remain on campus so that the university could do well in athletic events?

Recently administrative cover-ups on college campuses around student misconduct, especially sexual misconduct, have been nearly as egregious as the misconduct itself. Larry Nassar and Michigan State, Baylor's football program—in these instances, the institutional failures have put students at risk. The newspaper sought to hold its own institution accountable.

But no school wants to be the next Baylor. Is it any surprise that universities will use a highly complex law to block media inquiries? Sportswriter Jessica Luther, author of *Unsportsmanlike Conduct: College Football and the Politics of Rape* (Edge of Sports 2016), encounters pushback from universities under the guise of FERPA so frequently that she's taken to using FERPA as a verb: "I got FERPAed."

FERPA, though important for the protection of the privacy of our students, should not be a tool to protect the reputation of universities—at the expense of the students it is meant to protect.

17

PREDATORY PROFESSORS

When professors abuse their graduate students and get caught, they make higher education headlines. You can read about Jason Lieb, who stepped down from the University of Chicago, and Geoff Marcy, who did the same at the University of California at Berkeley. Both left their posts amid flurries of complaints by former graduate students and colleagues that the men had allegedly harassed, abused, and in one case, raped, graduate students. Few are defending these men.

But in other cases, the situations seem less clear-cut. The University of California-Riverside fired English professor Rob Latham in January of 2016, according to *Inside Higher Education*, "over alleged violations of the university's sexual harassment and drug and alcohol use policies." Debates raged on the American Association of University Professors *Academe* blog and other websites that featured the story, often focusing on the propriety of student-professor relationships in the first place. On one side, people have argued that policing relationships between graduate students and professors infantilizes graduate students. On the other, people have argued that the power imbalance in such relationships can blur the lines of consent.

I have my own story to tell. You might call it a story of blurred lines, perhaps, but the lines weren't blurry to me. I was terrified that I would be kicked out of my program because a professor wanted a sexual relationship with me and I turned him down. After I turned him down, after rumors started in the department that I was trying to seduce him, after his wife heard this rumors—I thought for sure that my career was over.

I'm lucky. I managed to get help from outside of the department and graduate without anyone standing in my way. The professor quickly moved on from me to start sleeping with a former undergraduate. Last I checked, he still had tenure.

―――

I HAVE one undergraduate degree and three graduate degrees. That makes me terminally educated. This is a story about one of those degrees. I will be vague on purpose to protect as many people as I can—including the professor's own family. This story takes place in a town with a university in it, one that I attended. The town could be Durham, Baltimore, Greensboro, or Chapel Hill.

The very worst part of this story is that it really could be any one of those towns: I have a similar story from all of them. In each of these towns, at each of these institutions, a professor I thought believed in me as a student, as a thinker, as a human, only wanted to get in my pants. Maybe he also thought I was smart—but he definitely wanted to get in my pants, too.

Each time it happened, I had the same terrible feeling when I realized I'd been duped. I had the same terrible feeling when I realized that my professors believed I only had one thing to contribute to the intellectual life of my community, and it had little to do with the intellectual life of my community.

All of the stories are terrible.

The worst of the stories is this one.

———

During the final months of my academic program, my serious boyfriend and I broke up. Newly single, I was dating, but not seriously. I was focusing on my work, not on anyone else's feelings.

Every Tuesday afternoon, the students in my program had a standing get-together at a cafe near campus. The cafe served coffee, of course, but it also served booze. Certain professors would often drop by. We graduate students all knew what that meant. They were looking to flirt, to feel young again, to get the student gossip.

I believed, hubristically, that I was above that sort of flirting. I believed I could see through these professors' nonsense. I was a very practical person, very direct, very plainspoken. Sometimes very bitchy. Usually, I was right.

But I had a weakness. I didn't want to be studying what I was studying. I wanted to be writing novels. I write novels now, but I didn't know then that I could. I thought I needed a "real job." I thought there was such a thing as a "real job." So I'd chosen a track that was more practical. At the cafe on Tuesdays, the poets sat together. The novelists sat together. And I sat alone at the bar, writing my novel and drinking Wild Turkey.

One Tuesday, a professor sat down next to me at the bar. I didn't know that this professor, with his speciality in fiction writing, would be able to charm me. I still believed I was beyond being charmed.

He ordered, gesturing at my glass. "Whatever she's having."

The bartender poured the Turkey, neat.

"Well." He assessed the beverage with admiration. "She'll be having another one. On me."

He didn't introduce himself. Didn't need to. Even though he wasn't in my area of study, he was still a senior member of my department. I knew who he was. He wrote books for a living. His job was to do what I wanted to do more than anything.

I set down my pen and finished the first glass of whiskey, pulling the second one closer. He lifted his in a toast. "To Tuesdays. And new friends."

"Isn't that a little over the top?"

"Maybe."

He wasn't physically attractive. Not in the slightest. He probably thought he was cool. He was charming, though, and he was smart. He was also a good writer—I'd been to his readings. Most importantly, though, he wanted to hang out with me. Not with the fiction kids sitting at their table. With me.

I made an error that many a university woman makes when a male professor pays attention to her outside the classroom. I believed he wanted to talk to me because he found me smart and interesting.

After our toast, we talked about breakups. I realize, now, that this part of the conversation might have raised red flags for some people. But we'd been talking about writing and work, and we were surrounded by other students. There didn't appear to be any danger. There didn't seem to be any reason for me to look for flags, red or otherwise. We discussed my recent breakup with my former boyfriend, and he mentioned he just been through one, too—he'd separated from his wife. I didn't examine his words closely, though, because I wasn't interested in him romantically. Who cared whether he was married. I certainly didn't. He was a professor, a novelist. I wanted to learn about the trade.

Starting that day, and over the course of some more afternoons, we became what I considered friends. We talked about writing, the novel I was laboring through with no guidance from anyone—from anyone besides him. We talked about his current projects. To me, we felt like colleagues.

I don't know what he thought we were.

———

AT THE TIME, I was living in a typical graduate school apartment with three other people. The apartment was little better than a flop-house, and we loved it. It was located walking distance from campus, which is all that really matters. The only thing more expensive than rent in a college town is parking. If this story were set in Baltimore, the area is Charles Village or Homewood; if this story were set in Durham, the area is Trinity Park; if this story were set in Greensboro, the area is College Park; if this story were set in Chapel Hill, the area is Westwood or Cameron-McCauley. You get the idea. Every college town has its just off-campus neighborhoods, its apartments where students cram themselves tight to save money on expenses and, perhaps, to stave off loneliness.

One night, after a departmental event, the professor invited himself back to the apartment. I didn't think anything of it. I had three roommates. I thought he wanted to hang out with us. It would be just like the Tuesday afternoon café gatherings. What was going to happen?

When we got to my apartment, though, no one else was home. So the professor and I sat in my living room and talked. We ate cheese.

After about twenty minutes, he jumped to his feet and ran to the far side of the room. "Oh my god," he whispered.

"What?"

"I think that's my wife outside."

Through the curtains, the professor had spied the headlights of his wife's car, parked on the street. "I thought you were separated?" I yelled. To myself, I thought: *Where are my roommates? Why is no one here with me?* I was distraught about my terrible luck.

"We're separated, but we're still living together." He sounded small. He looked small. And he looked like a coward.

"That means you are not separated, you idiot," I spat. Then I kicked him out of my apartment.

And then, once I'd locked the door, I started to worry about my future in my academic program.

The next day, a friend told me why the professor's wife ended up outside my apartment. One of the professor's students had seen him leave the school event with me. The student had called his wife at home and told her where he'd gone. The caller had speculated about why he'd gone to my apartment. The speculations had been inaccurate, but they'd been enough to send his wife after her husband.

She'd been watching us through the curtains in my living room. For a while. She'd seen nothing, of course, except two people talking. It didn't matter what she'd seen. His wife was really angry with me. Really, really angry.

The speculations had also started rumors. That I was breaking up a marriage. That I was a seducer of professors. That I was a slut. That I was a troublemaker. And it wasn't just students that heard these rumors. Other professors did too.

I still needed to graduate and get references for jobs. This man's colleagues were my gatekeepers. How many of them were friends with his wife? How many of them were angry enough with me to stand in my way?

AT THE TIME, I was not angry at the professor's wife for being mad at me. I would have been angry at me, too. She thought I was breaking up her marriage. I wasn't, but she didn't know that. I placed the blame on his shoulders completely—on his, and those of the rumormongers.

And today, I'm certainly not angry at his wife for being

angry at me. Since this incident occurred, I've gotten married and had two children. I know what lengths I would go to to protect my family.

At the time, though, I was scared of her, just like I was scared of him. I feared for my diploma. I worried that either he or his wife would stand in the way of my graduation and job prospects afterward. I didn't know what to do. I didn't know what they would do to me.

The next day, while I was out of the apartment, I got a phone call from one of my roommates. "Something weird just happened. This woman came to the door with her kid."

I knew what she was going to say next. I just knew.

"She said, 'Are you Kate?' And I laughed, because, you know, we look nothing alike."

I tried to laugh too, and failed.

"I said no. But it's like she didn't believe me. She said, 'I have children!' And she pulled her kid in front of her and said, 'This is my child!' It was weird."

I could barely breathe. "Then what?"

"She made me write down a note for you. I have it here. It has her name on it, and her phone number. I think she wants you to call her."

I asked, "What kind of car was she driving?" I needed to know who was after me.

She didn't know what I looked like, and I didn't know what she looked like. It felt like she was an unknown assassin and I was her unknown target.

I was truly terrified—all of my hard work and all of my student loans, they would be for nothing. He had all of the power, and I had none. He wasn't even in my field, but that didn't matter—I knew that all of the negative consequences would fall on me. I was an expendable student. He was a tenured professor.

When I should have been working on my studies, I was worrying about whether I needed to protect myself legally.

When I couldn't take the worry anymore, I consulted an attorney.

The entire time I sat in the attorney's office, I felt humiliated. The man was very fatherly, and respectable, and kind. And there I was, telling him about this ugly fake-love-triangle that I was caught in the middle of. I was Hester Prynne. I was dirty. I cried. I couldn't help it. "Can he stop me from graduating?"

"No way." He sounded very certain.

"How do you know?"

"I know."

"I'm so embarrassed," I admitted.

He looked surprised. "Why? Do you honestly think you're the first student he's tried this on?"

No, I realized. I did not think I was the first student he'd tried this on.

For the first time since the headlights appeared outside my apartment that awful night, I started to relax.

The lawyer helped me make a plan. He gave me his mobile number, and he told me to call him if either the professor or his wife approached me again. "Let me handle it." I knew I was lucky that I had the means to consult a lawyer.

I'VE since found out that the professor slept with young female students on a regular basis. I know of two young women from that one year alone. One sexual relationship had ended right before he took aim at me, and one began right after me. The reason his marriage ended was because of an affair with a girl younger than I was. His wife had found suspicious credit card receipts.

But here's the deal, the worst part of it all: I had been afraid that I would get in trouble for turning down the advances of a tenured professor, for false rumors, as there were many of those. I was terrified, yet absolutely nothing had happened between him and me.

But what if I'd been a little more vulnerable, or a little attracted to him? What if I'd kissed him? What if I'd slept with him, believing him to be separated or divorced? Then what? Would that have made me? Would I have deserved the scorn and trouble? Would I have deserved censure by my department? Would I have deserved to have my own advisors turn their backs on me for hurting their friend, his wife? Would that have made me the seductress, the slut, like the rumormongers insisted?

Or was he a predator, like my lawyer said?

Of course he was. A predator with lifetime job security and easy access to prey.

18

METOO COMES TO CAMPUS
CAN WE STOP SEXUAL HARASSMENT IN HIGHER ED?

During my higher education experiences, like many (if not most) of my women colleagues, I was sexually harassed by male professors. As I describe in the previous chapter of this book, I feared for my career, my grades, my friendships. The men suffered no consequences. I walked around campus (each campus) panicked, terrified of what might happen to me, terrified of who was my enemy or my friend. I didn't realize until years later how traumatizing these experiences were. Or how normal. I blamed myself. After all, why did these men keep approaching me? It must be my fault, right?

I now know that it wasn't my fault. I also know that they didn't only approach me. But when you keep harassment to yourself like a secret shame, then you don't know who else is suffering as you are. But for those who are harassed on campus, there is little incentive to come forward about our harassment. The men (and it is mostly men) who are our supervisors and senior colleagues so rarely suffer consequences.

The #MeToo movement sought to change that by supporting survivors of sexual abuse and harassment. With that support, many of us came forward. Some of us named names. And with these survivors coming forward en masse, men suddenly faced consequences for their actions.

In November of 2017, comics author and publisher Charlie "Spike" Trotman wrote on Twitter: "God, I could really get used to this strange new world of Men Experiencing Consequences." She hit on two points that rang horribly true to the thousands of readers who made her tweet go viral: (1) men were experiencing real consequences for harming others (2) for the first time in U.S. historical memory. Harvey Weinstein, the most powerful man in Hollywood, lost his company. Kevin Spacey, megastar, lost his hit television show. Charlie Rose, highly respected broadcaster, lost his contracts. The abusive kings were tumbling from their thrones for the first time that any of us could remember, or even imagine.

After decades (centuries, millennia) of Hollywood and other powerful entities turning their eyes away from abusers and rapists or even celebrating them (e.g., Woody Allen, Roman Polanski, Thomas Jefferson, ad nauseam), it seems that things are finally changing.

I thought of my own experiences in my career, higher education: How are these changes translating to academia? Are we seeing similar changes there? Is there similar support for victims and survivors by colleagues and faculty? Is there similar institutional support for those who come forward?

Right now, it doesn't look like it. As legal expert Caroline Fredrickson wrote for the Atlantic, it doesn't look like the "Harvey Effect" is going to hit higher ed any time soon. Why? As she explains in "When Will the 'Harvey Effect' Reach Academia?" (October 2017), male professors dominate the upper echelons of academia, and they hold an immense amount of largely unchecked power over the careers of graduate students and junior faculty. Consequently, "[w]hen an adviser or a prominent professor puts his hand on his younger colleague's thigh or asks a graduate mentee to come talk to him in his hotel room at a conference, this woman knows too well the consequences of saying no." For all of these reasons, Frederickson explains, "Academia is particularly fertile territory for those who want to leverage their power to gain sexual favors or inflict sexual violence on vulnerable individuals."

I experienced these imbalances of power first-hand. I escaped relatively unscathed. But I didn't know how to stop these same men from hurting others.

I spoke to a woman colleague recently, one who works in higher education, about an informational panel she attended for women students about how to handle sexual harassment. The panel was led by women faculty, although some male faculty were in attendance as audience members. One woman student asked the panel about what to do when harassed while working an internship. What was the best response? What did the panelists recommend?

The women faculty on the panel said, unanimously, "There really isn't a good answer to that question." The panelists then recognized the difficulty in figuring out the proper response to sexual harassment, especially when working a hard-to-get internship.

Before the panelists could expand on their responses, a

male faculty member in the audience spoke up. He said, "You can report harassment to Human Resources. That's the most aggressive move. The least aggressive is just telling the harasser in the moment that his actions are inappropriate."

As my friend told me this story, we were overwhelmed by how wrong this male faculty member's advice was. His "least aggressive move" was confronting a harasser in the moment? He couldn't fathom that a confrontation such as that is actually incredibly aggressive. And yet, every victim of harassment knows that it is. To make a ruckus in the workplace draws attention to the victim, not to the harasser. Harassment tends to be subtle. It's a "joke." To cause a scene—well, you've caused a scene. Now, you're the problem. Not him. Survivors of harassment know that harassers use this precise double-bind to harass with impunity.

Instead, survivors know the other strategies we must use. How to make the soothing smile. How to speak the appeasing words. How to make a quick escape without being harmed further.

But this male faculty member's advice—to a room full of women students—reveals a larger problem. Senior men in academia (some men) do not understand the peril, and attendant fear, that all women face, all of the time, including in academia. And as study after study of sexual violence against men show, although men are less likely to experience sexual violence than women, they are even less likely to report than women for fear that they won't be believed.

Senior men in academia do not understand the

appeasing all women must do of men for even the most basic job retention, let alone promotion, whether we are graduate students, faculty members, or staff. Beyond appeasement, we must ignore all kinds of harassment. We don't have a choice. What that young, female student was asking was not how to make the harassment stop—she was asking how to make her life with a harasser just a little less awful.

When I was teaching at one of my many institutions, a senior male faculty member approached a group of female graduate students when they greeted him. I was standing to the side, outside my classroom, just before my class began. They spoke to him about a surgery he'd had a while back. While I watched, he raised his shirt, baring his chest, to, as he said, *show his scars*. The female students grew obviously uncomfortable—to my well-trained eyes—although the male faculty member seemed not to notice. And then he ambled off. I dashed into my classroom and shut the door. I did nothing. What could I say? And to whom? The questions raced in my head.

What if one of the students had said to him, in that moment, to put his clothes back on, that his nudity made her uncomfortable—if she'd confronted him? Look into your heart—you know the answer. I knew it too, at the time. In that hallway, in that building, with other professors and students in classrooms and offices, her voice would have been the one causing a scene, a ruckus. She would have been the troublemaker. Not him.

It was easier for those students to smile weakly, to let him do what he came to do, and never speak of it again.

And for me, an untenured woman faculty member—it was easier for me to do the same.

Remember Harvey Weinstein's most famous victims? These are women who hold incredible power—in their own right, but also because of their formidable family legacies. Angelina Jolie didn't go public or confront anyone, and her dad is Jon ("Deliverance") Voight. Gwyneth Paltrow didn't either, and her mom is Blythe ("I have 250 Tony Awards") Danner. Mira Sorvino didn't, and her dad is Paul ("Goodfellas") Sorvino. Ashley Judd didn't, and she's a Judd. If these powerhouse members of powerhouse families didn't think it was worth it to go public, to go to HR or to the courts, why would anyone? After all, it wasn't like Jolie, Paltrow, Sorvino, Judd, or any of the rest were going to end up in the poorhouse, right?

But some of Harvey's victims did go public, and they did suffer, and they did lose their careers.

What the Harvey stories should teach us is that women, no matter how powerful, learn to appease. To give the calming smile. To coddle harassers, and then, later, to warn other women in secret. After that professor took off his shirt in front of those students, I texted a female colleague and told her what happened. That's what we so often have to do—we whisper, we warn, and we hope it's enough.

But sometimes we have a chance to do more, a chance like this book or some column inches in a magazine. And when we have a chance like that, some of us do more. We speak loudly about what happened, and what might happen if more people don't act. We know that we're taking a risk by speaking up. Even if the risk is relatively small, it's a risk nonetheless. We take that risk.

And we say to others who have a loud voice like ours: *You, you need to say something, too. Otherwise nothing will ever change.*

You. Please. Say something, too.

NOTES

3. Being Counted

1. Shelley Ng, "College student could be expelled for reporting her rape and creating an 'intimidating environment' for her alleged rapist," *New York Daily News*, February 27, 2013.
2. The Jeanne Clery Disclosure of Campus Security Policy and Campus Crime Statistics Act, also called simply the Clery Act, is a federal law that requires colleges that accept federal financial aid to report all crimes that occur on campus or near campus, within what is called a campus's "Clery Geography." Universities tend to be super conscious about whether a crime is within its Clery Geography because they do not want the crime on the university record if it is not—even if the crime occurred in a common student hangout.

8. Nightmare Room

1. *Dulieu v. White & Sons*, 2 K.B. 669 (High Court King's Bench), 1901.

ACKNOWLEDGMENTS

This book was made possible with the help of many people and organizations.

I thank my friend-editors and readers: Lauren Faulkenberry, fellow writer, my primary editor, and my writing partner. Alexa Chew and Gentry Hodnett, early readers of this book. Tamiya Anderson, intern at Blue Crow Books.

I thank my supportive community of fellow writers: Kelly J. Baker, fellow writer and my editor at *Women in Higher Education*. Virginia C. McGuire, fellow writer and an early writing mentor. Catherine Prendergast, fellow academic, rabble-rouser, and writer.

I thank Kelly Harms, who read the final proof of this book and told me to publish it because it didn't suck, and Camille Pagán, who read it after it came out and reminded me that it didn't suck. (That's what I heard in my head, but they probably used better words. They always use better words.)

I thank the incredible community of activists and

writers that have supported and guided me over the years: Andrea Pino, Annie Clark, and Jessica Luther. Sydette Harry, fellow writer and activist, to whom I dedicate the chapter "Nightmare Room," especially. (You're the only one who gets a whole chapter to herself.)

Some of these chapters first appeared as essays, in whole or in part—and heavily edited since—in various publications over the years. I owe these publications and their editors deep thanks: "Why Birds Have Wings," a short story, in *Bayou Magazine*. "Why I Didn't Report Being Raped" in *Side B Magazine*, edited by Morgan Jerkins. "Being Counted" and "Predatory Professors" in *The Toast*, edited by Nicole Cliffe and Nicole Chung. "Over Nothing" in *The Chronicle of Higher Education*, edited by Gabriela Montell and Denise Magner. "Even If You're Broken" in *The Huffington Post*. "Reading Romance When You Were Never a Virgin" in *Full Grown People* edited by Jennifer Niesslein. "How to Write Publicly About Rape," "Handling Institutional Atrocities," "So Many Brett Kavanaughs," "Banning College Athletes for Sexual Assault Convictions is Not Enough," "Why We Should All Care About FERPA," and "MeToo Comes to Campus," in *Women in Higher Education*, edited by Kelly J. Baker. "Why Kesha Lost" in *DAME Magazine*, edited by Kera Bolonik and Jennifer Reitman, "How Campus Rape Changed Mental Health Privacy for All," a fusion of essays from *DAME Magazine* and *Women in Higher Ed*, and "Cosby and Rethinking Statutes of Limitations" in *Quartz*, edited by Meredith Bennett-Smith.

I thank my local community, including Annie Johnston and Erin Pacheco of La Vita Dolce in Chapel Hill, NC. If I can ever hold a launch party for this book, I will hold it there.

I thank the Orange County Rape Crisis Center for the important work that they do in our community, and for being there for me many years ago when I needed them.

And finally: My husband and children, fellow creatures with hearts that can break, and then mend, fiercely.

ABOUT THE AUTHOR

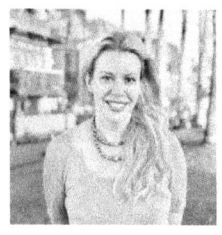

Katie Rose Guest Pryal, J.D., Ph.D., is an award-winning author, speaker, and professor of law and creative writing.

She is the author of *Life of the Mind Interrupted: Essays on Mental Health and Disability in Higher Education* (2017), a #1 Amazon bestseller; *The Freelance Academic: Transform Your Creative Life and Career* (2019), winner of a Gold INDIE award; and *Even If You're Broken: Essays on Sexual Assault and #MeToo* (2019), winner of a Gold IPPY award. She is also the author of novels, which include *Entanglement*, *Chasing Chaos*, and *Fallout Girl*.

Her short pieces have appeared in *Catapult*, *Women in Higher Education*, *Dame Magazine*, *The Toast*, *The Chronicle of Higher Education,* and more.

She lives in Chapel Hill, North Carolina, with her spouse, children, and many, many animals. Visit her website and blog, where you can read stories about her life, at katieroseguestpryal.com.

She writes a monthly email letter about writing, creativity, and more, "Words Can Change the World," and you can subscribe at pryalnews.com.

- facebook.com/krgpryal
- twitter.com/krgpryal
- instagram.com/krgpryal
- amazon.com/author/krgp
- bookbub.com/authors/katie-rose-guest-pryal
- goodreads.com/krgpryal

CPSIA information can be obtained
at www.ICGtesting.com
Printed in the USA
LVHW050450180722
723716LV00003B/355